Dance
of the
Dragonfly

Dance of the Dragonfly

GETTING SOBER BROUGHT ME
PURPOSE AND ALLOWED ME TO
BECOME MY OWN BEST FRIEND

DANIELLE EHLERT

ISBN: 978-1-958150-67-2
Dance of the Dragonfly: Getting Sober Brought Me Purpose and Allowed Me to Become My Own Best Friend

First edition: August 29, 2025

Published by Inner Peace Press
Eau Claire, Wisconsin, USA
www.innerpeacepress.com

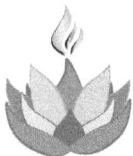

Dedication

I dedicate this book to my husband and best friend, Bryon Ehlert. He has proven his love for me time and time again. He has stood strong during many challenging times in our 32-year relationship and remained my anchor through difficulties I thought I could never overcome. His belief in our love never wavered. What could have torn us apart only made us stronger. Thanks to his heroic effort when I had my cardiac arrest, I am able to tell my story today. He made it possible by breathing for me when he found me unresponsive. He attended every doctor's appointment, serving as my memory. He helped with the children when I couldn't due to physical or mental health issues. He held everything together while I battled alcoholism and healed from a lifetime of trauma. He stood by me as I unraveled after the deaths of my parents, my beloved grandmother, and my sister. He was there when I was admitted to a psych hospital after a bad reaction to an antidepressant. He never judged me – he took it all in stride. My husband is a mechanic and is the hardest worker I know. Reserved by nature, he doesn't voice opinions often or share his struggles. He's not college educated, but he's the smartest person I've ever met. He epitomizes love and patience. He's a brilliant father, a loyal nurse with a lovely bedside manner, and a capable man who can do anything he sets his mind to. He has helped me back from the brink of death more than once – literally and figuratively. This book is my thank you to him for everything he has done. *Dance of the Dragonfly* symbolizes what can happen when you believe in yourself. Thank you, Bryon, for always believing in this dragonfly!

Table of Contents

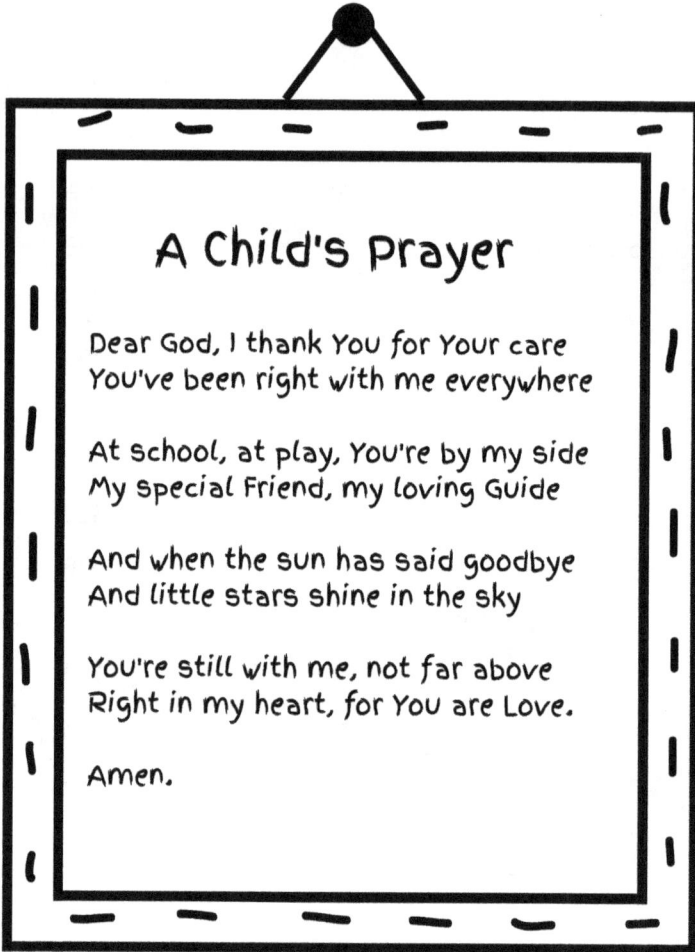

A Child's Prayer

Dear God, I thank You for Your care
You've been right with me everywhere

At school, at play, You're by my side
My special Friend, my loving Guide

And when the sun has said goodbye
And little stars shine in the sky

You're still with me, not far above
Right in my heart, for You are Love.

Amen.

Introduction

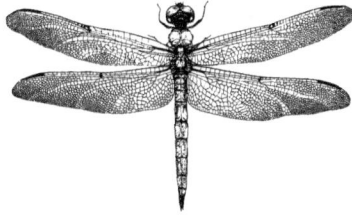

During my journey here on Earth I have witnessed myself go through a sort of metamorphosis. Similar to that of a dragonfly transforming from an egg, into a nymph, to finally shedding its familiar shell to evolve into the beautiful dragonfly. I reflect on the process of its evolution. Each of us has to go through a similar process. It's a painful, complicated journey of learning to love ourselves.

Dragonflies have been around for centuries. They have become a symbol of strength and resilience for many. While my journey has not been easy, I now understand it was all part of the process of becoming the person I am today. The person I was created to be. I respect and honor the struggle of growth. It's necessary for each of us to understand who we are and why we are the way we are today. It's a self inventory of sorts. Checking in with ourselves to see if the beliefs we hold onto so diligently are actually in our best interest. Often it is surprising to realize that some of those beliefs are the very things that keep us stuck and unfulfilled. The dragonfly needed to shed its shell to grow, I needed to shed my beliefs about myself.

I realized that I believed for far too long that I was unlovable and unworthy of happiness. It was the dialogue I had with myself for so many years... Not good enough. Too much for others. Too sensitive. Misunderstood. And worse. I didn't know how to love myself at all. I kept trying to live up to everyone else's expectations of me and in doing so I didn't know who I really was. I needed to believe in myself. I needed to prove myself to myself to make a change.

Like the dragonfly that emerges from the mud and sludge when born and grabs onto the reed, believing in something greater, I was determined to find myself. Though it wasn't easy, it has been a very rewarding endeavor. I am no longer fearful of life. For too many years I avoided taking risks or stepping out of my comfort zone. I played small so I would not bother or offend anyone. My advice to you is to believe in yourself. Take chances in life. Challenge yourself. Hold yourself accountable, but do so understanding that by design we are all imperfect creatures. Give yourself and others grace. Understand that everyone is dealing with their own problems. We are all just doing the best we know how. Once we know better, we do better. It's that simple. So always be kind. Especially to yourself.

Ironically the lifespan of the dragonfly is very short – on average they only live two or three weeks. As humans we average around 72 short years. Today I am 56 and I already survived a near death experience. I understand how quickly my time here on Earth is diminishing. I have already been given 21 bonus years, and I remain grateful for each and every day. It has become my mission to live in the present and make the most of the things that come my way. I live with gratitude knowing it could have ended much differently. I practice kindness when needed and give myself and others grace. *Dance of the Dragonfly* is about loving and understanding the person I am becoming. It's about embracing sobriety and letting go of beliefs and people who no longer serve me so I can become the best version of myself.

During my healing process I was very lonely. I realized that I often showed up for people who never reciprocated when I was struggling. As an empath (a term I've only recently come to truly understand), I've always had a perspective that others failed to understand. I see now that my empathy for others was a gift as I knew what it felt like to be them. My friends had no awareness of how I felt, and few ever made any attempt to understand our differences. I needed more from friends than idle chit chat. I yearned to be with others who strive to become the best versions of themselves. I needed more than phony, backstabbing, superficial friends. I longed for a much deeper connection with people. Although I deeply cared about so many people, I felt guided to move on. It took me years and so much drama to finally accept this about myself and to make the change I needed in my life.

Now I know my worth. I understand that not everyone is meant to accompany me on my journey these days. I understand that they no longer deserve my loyalty. I no longer hold space for them in my life. With no hard feelings, I wish them well. I know that God is making a way for the right people to come into my life today. People who inspire and empower me. People living their best lives, helping one another.

Establishing boundaries was the biggest answer for me to make change. Establishing new boundaries is guaranteed to be difficult, but it is a necessary process. Consistency is crucial. I'd tried to implement boundaries, but never followed through or stood my ground. Without addressing these boundary issues I grew angry and resentful. I also realized they were the main reason I had sabotaged my sobriety in the past. It was easier to just go back to the way things had always been instead of enforcing my boundaries.

There was a lot of resistance from my children and husband. Even though I've always been "a lot," I'd never really asserted myself much before I was sober. I used alcohol as a coping mechanism for most of my life, so being sober and trying to keep my desired boundaries was a daunting task for me. Old feelings and emotions flooded my mind. I addressed many of these things in therapy. I realized that

I had been living as a victim due to my illnesses. After my cardiac arrest I *became* my heart disease. When they found the mass on my liver I *became* my liver disease. The nodules in my lungs from years of smoking led me to believe I had lung cancer. Then I stumbled across two transformational thought leaders: Joe Dispenza and Gregg Braden. I learned about the Law of Attraction – how our thoughts become our reality. These men explained quantum physics in a way that I could understand. I started to visualize what it would feel like to be happy and healthy. I learned that with the right perspective, nothing is impossible. I prayed for guidance. I started visualizing myself being healthy and happy. I tried to act as if it were already a reality. Slowly I started to notice that I wasn't quite as sore, or quite as sad as I had been. I noticed the more I practiced these techniques, the happier I felt. I visualized myself dancing gracefully and with ease. Despite years of self loathing, during this process I fell in love with myself. My life started to change.

Remarkably, while streaming YouTube videos, I discovered some motivational speakers who inspired me. I started my days listening to encouraging and uplifting videos. I put into practice techniques of how to stay motivated in my daily routine. It became important for me to practice gratitude daily. An attitude of gratitude is a worthwhile endeavor. You must simply choose to notice the wonderful things in your life each day. The simple things you will find will bring you great joy.

I challenge you to give it a try. Look for three things that you are grateful for and write them down daily. You will find that you truly have so much to be grateful for. Happiness comes from within. Look within yourself to reveal what truly brings you joy in life. Doing an inventory of your life will really bring things into perspective. We have an abundance right in front of us that most people only dream of. When one is appreciative, the universe will bring you even more to be grateful for. That is how I came to understand the Law of Attraction. It is the real deal.

Like many, I've had a complicated relationship with God throughout my life. But this period of learning helped me see that it was God who answered all of my prayers. All my life all I had ever wanted was a family that loved me. Thankfully my prayers were answered when Bryon entered my life. I couldn't have asked for a more perfect husband. Together now for 32 years, I can't imagine my life without him. I am mindful of how time is flying by each day. I live for each day together with him. I thank God for bringing us together every day. *Amor fati*, I am thankful for all of it – the highs and lows, the good and bad, all of it. My prayers were answered even when I felt unworthy and unlovable. God made it possible.

Most of my friends agree that I am the most stubborn person they have ever encountered. I'm not sure if it is meant to be a compliment, but I take it as such. I am not easily swayed on my opinions, however I try to stay open to new ideas. I understand just how little I know about life. God, however, has revealed that I am needed. It's through my own experiences that I have empathy for others who are struggling. By sharing my stories it is my hope that someone may have a different perspective that they hadn't experienced before. It may be the inspiration they need to tackle their own beliefs and ideas that no longer serve them. I know that's what it took for me... I have met some truly inspirational individuals. When I believed I was too old to make new friends, God opened doors for me and I now feel empowered by other people.

I have hope for the future for those of us who are struggling. I want to start the dialogue and normalize healing from trauma and addiction. No more shame or guilt. This has become my passion. I feel like this is what God is guiding me to do. I am filled these days with His Love. Every day I serve others and I am truly blessed. God brings the right people into my life so I am able to create new and beautiful friendships.

God healed my physical ailments. My heart disease has improved. My heart is functioning like a well trained athlete. Just recently, after a couple years of being off blood pressure medicine, I had to return to taking a low dose blood pressure medicine during a very stressful time. I am determined to regain the balance in my life necessary to get off of it very soon. I really believe in using natural remedies these days.

The mass in my liver resolved itself. One of my many miracles from God. I didn't understand how remarkable it was for this to happen until my doctor explained that people with a liver mass rarely were discharged from hepatology. This was an answered prayer and I knew it.

The nodules in my lungs are believed to be debris from a faulty CPAP device – not only from my smoking for 36 years. They were not lung cancer as I had feared. God gave me another chance to breathe freely. He made quitting cigarettes possible without drugs, or hypnosis. He gifted me with pure strong-willed intention to quit. I also believe that in my quitting cigarettes, I was able to fulfill something both my parents and my sister couldn't. It made me very proud to have recently celebrated five years off cigarettes.

Due to my past, I will most likely always have some sort of health issues, but I give myself grace these days, especially having learned that many diseases can be attributed to trauma. I am a living testament of how trauma manifests into illness, even later in life, if not dealt with. My heart physically stopped 21 years ago, at age 35. I believe it was because I had survived by living in fight or flight mode for most of my life. My body was responding to the overwhelm and exhaustion of not being true to myself. I believe that by trying to be accepted by others I lost sight of myself. Today I am able to be authentic to myself. I live my life with integrity and a desire to be of service to others.

My illnesses forced me to slow down and evaluate life. To face my demons. To deal with generations of dysfunction that ran through my family's lineage. To take ownership of my faults and shortcomings. To discover my strengths and know my weaknesses. I needed to understand why I was the way I was. Why are we here? It certainly wasn't just to work and pay taxes. There had to be more to all the suffering and I wanted to understand. By surrendering myself to God, I came to understand unconditional love for us as humans. I started to let go of my need to control everything. I began to research natural healing techniques. I took control of my life and started to heal naturally, as God intended.

I now understand that there are demonic forces trying to keep us from God. I have witnessed some of the worst in humanity. In instances when I have been hurt or betrayed by someone, I now work towards forgiveness over revenge. Seeking revenge kept me stuck. I was able to give that burden to God to deal with. Only then was I free to move forward. I had to forgive those who I would never receive closure or apologies from. I was set free from that longing for them to experience the pain they had caused me. I instantly felt lighter and was able to breathe easily again.

For years I went against what my little-girl-self imagined: that I would not smoke or drink, because I understood at a young age that it was toxic. I didn't know about the health side of it as I do now, but I knew the hurt I felt from the constant let-downs and lack of nurturing from my own parents, and family. Despite my own desires, I ended up going down the route of self numbing. Cocaine, marijuana, speed, and alcohol in my teenage years throughout high school. Adulthood brought the benzos. The seemingly never-ending pain I experienced made life too hard to face sober. Over the years I'd made multiple attempts at sobriety, and each time failed. Even after the losses of people I loved, I kept avoiding what I now embrace: putting myself first and learning how to love myself, and finding acceptance so I didn't need the "pain relievers." Though finding God nearly killed me, I'm now doing things I had only dreamed of before.

I have come to understand that hurt people hurt people. I was guilty of hurting others. While it was never my intention, it happened. I have since owned up to my faults and shortcomings. I acknowledge my imperfections, and I take steps to be aware of how I treat others. I practice kindness everyday. If I see a need, I do what I can to help. I know I can't fix everything, but God is capable of miracles! I am proof that He can work miracles. He brought me hope when I was hopeless. He gave me strength to persevere. He healed my heart from despair. He filled me with love and self acceptance. He revealed my purpose and restored my life with joy. I am eternally grateful for His mercy and grace.

Overcoming many challenges throughout my life helped me to develop resilience. By reexamining and nurturing my beliefs about God I was able to see that those challenges were actually blessings. Navigating the depths of Hell in my mind to learn to actually love myself was only possible with

God's grace. This is my story of recovery from years of addiction and mental illness. I had to heal myself physically, emotionally, and spiritually. I am now helping others who are struggling. I share how forgiveness set me free. Surrendering my burdens to God allowed closure for some things I could never let go of. He replaced fear and unworthiness with forgiveness and love. I went from sick and hopeless to a heart filled with joy and purpose. It's my sincere hope that my story will encourage you to reconnect with your spiritual beliefs, to find your purpose, and to live a life filled with joy and empathy for others.

God is giving me strength to speak up for others who are unable to speak up for themselves. Through writing poems or telling my story at events I hope to bring about awareness and compassion for others. God's grace makes it possible. He can help you too. I encourage others to invite God into their lives. I do not think I would be writing this without His guidance today in my life. His healing love is responsible for me being able to share my story of hope with others.

Dance of the Dragonfly is my story of learning to love myself. I have learned I am much stronger than I believed and that I have a lot to offer others. While change is very scary, it is needed to grow. Self acceptance must come from within. Love yourself enough to work on it. Look for the lessons. Our creator thought of everything. He gave us the tools and rules for life. When you surrender yourself to God, your life will change in ways you haven't even imagined. I never thought I would become a writer, yet here I am. I never imagined I would be able to work again. Now I am a caregiver and storyteller. We often hold ourselves back because of fear of failure. We tell ourselves things that keep us living in limbo. We hold tightly to our beliefs and refuse to change. We blame our unhappiness on our circumstances and allow our job, parents, health, and family to dictate who we are. We have to inventory our own lives and take steps to become the best version of ourselves. What do you want to accomplish for yourself? Dare to be your best self! You will be amazed at what you can accomplish. The sky's the limit once you believe in yourself.

Dear reader, I give you *Dance of the Dragonfly*, my memoir of overcoming childhood trauma, alcoholism, and severe health challenges, while understanding my relationship with the universe – and myself. Namaste.

Danielle Ehlert
August 2025
Arena, Wisconsin

My Story

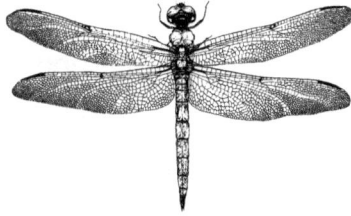

I was born into a dysfunctional family. My father was a professional baseball player who played for several teams during his 17 year career; he was best known for getting the Baltimore Orioles to the 1966 World Series against the New York Yankees. He did not pitch the series due to an injury, but he got them into the series. He was eventually inducted into the Orioles Hall of Fame back in 1988.

I was born in September of 1968, just six weeks before my mother's father passed away. My mother decided to leave me with my grandmother just weeks after I was born. She claimed she thought it would help Grandma endure the loss of her husband. I believe she wanted to be on the road with my father and didn't want to take care of me. Her "freedom" didn't last long, though, because she became pregnant with my sister within weeks of my birth. Tracy was born the following June.

We were nine months and two days apart. I know... somebody couldn't wait!

While my father pursued his baseball career we moved around a lot and I lived in Florida, Georgia, Arizona, California, and Nevada. Every year we spent three months in the summer at the 113-acre farm in Wisconsin with Grandma. In the Fall she would return to Arizona or Nevada and winter with us. My parents used her as a built-in babysitter during these times. Other times we were left in the care of babysitters or others who brought trauma into our lives. From an early age we endured things that children should never have to experience. We were then threatened to never speak about what happened or things would really get worse.

A friend of my grandma's, named Don, used to bounce me on his knees when I was very young. I remembered him grooming me by massaging his fingers between my legs. It gave me a funny feeling, but I didn't understand why.

My sister would celebrate her birthday every year at the farm. On my sister's ninth birthday, my aunt Marie was visiting. She was a mean alcoholic. At the party my aunt and I got into a fight about something. I left the party to take a walk and cool off. I hated Aunt Marie. We were like oil and water. She always liked Tracy over me. I always felt like she was gunning for me, but never knew why. My dog, Pepper, and I headed out towards the barn. I heard someone coming up from behind me. It was Don. He asked if he could join me. I said sure. We headed into the pasture and past the barn. Don grabbed me from behind and started to molest me. He jammed his hand down my pants and tried penetrating me. I fought him off and ran back to the house with Pepper. Don followed. I ran upstairs and started crying. What had just happened? I was in shock. Aunt Marie came upstairs to see why I wasn't back at the party. She saw me crying and wanted to know why. I told her what Don had done. She ordered me to get into the bathtub, assuring me it would help me to feel better. I did as she ordered. I sat in the tub for what seemed to be an hour. I still felt dirty. As I drained the tub I felt my innocence disappear with the water.

Aunt Marie told Grandma what I had told her. Grandma became unhinged, saying what a filthy little girl I was. The next morning she drove me to Don's gas station to speak with him and his wife about my accusations. Though I was only nine years old, I stood my ground and repeated the story to him and his wife. Of course he denied everything. They were convinced that I made it all up. Grandma figured I had seen something between my parents and that had to be where I had gotten the idea. I, of course, was the liar, not Don. He and Grandma remained friends. In fact she often visited them with me in the car. I prayed that karma would visit Don. I grew to hate him and his nasty smile. I became hell-bent on seeking revenge for what he had done to me. I have since learned that it was a colossal waste of time and energy. My feelings regarding Don eventually became a wedge between me and my grandma. I never felt like I could tell her anything about what was happening in my life ever again. She broke my heart by remaining his friend.

Shortly after my now-husband Bryon and I started dating, I received a call from a woman claiming to be Don's granddaughter in Texas. She somehow tracked me down to find out what Don had done to me years earlier. Her grandmother, Florence, Don's wife, had relayed the story of a little girl named Danielle who had accused him of molesting her years ago. Unfortunately the granddaughter only learned about this after catching Don molesting her own infant daughter, ironically also named Danielle. The rage I felt inside of me exploded. He could've and should've been stopped after what he did to me, but no one would listen. The story of my life was that no one ever listened to me. No one saved me and now another child was victimized. His granddaughter promised me that she would be prosecuting him to the full extent allowed by the law. I never heard back from her. Again, no closure.

I experienced the feelings of the event every time I thought about that day. I had prayed for him to pay for his crimes. I wanted him to suffer as I had suffered silently for so many years. It saddened me that this event came between me and my grandmother. Nothing could resolve the resentment I carried for her for remaining his friend. My grandma and I never talked about what Don did to me. It changed how I saw her. She didn't want to know the truth. I never disclosed anything of substance to her ever again. Instead I learned to numb myself with alcohol to kill the pain from her betrayal.

I returned to Las Vegas that fall, when I was 9, turning 10. My parents always treated me like I was older than I was, yet they were nervous about the types of people I might meet in Vegas, so as an incentive to be "good" they promised me when we moved there that if I got good grades and avoided the wrong crowds that they would buy me a horse. My father left to go to Hawaii for a celebrity golf tournament. My mom drove me out to a ranch to see a horse for sale. Dandy was a 4-year-old registered Paint broodmare. She was absolutely gorgeous. I fell head over heels in love. We boarded her at a ranch close to our home. I made many friends at the ranch. I spent all my free time with Dandy. She became my confidant and best friend. I started training in gymkhana and dreamed of us competing in the rodeo circuit someday. My dream of having my own horse had finally come true! I realize now that Dandy was a stand in for a therapist my parents should have gotten me.

I was going to be starting middle school. It was a tough age. It is hard for anyone at that age, but add in my family's issues, it was even worse. My parents had been fighting a lot because of my mother's gambling. Every night was a drunken fiasco. My mom was always ornery and stressed about money. She was shuffling money between accounts trying to avoid overdraft fees and hide how bad things had gotten. Dad was defeated and would drink until he passed out nightly.

Dysfunction, lies, and betrayal abounded. It was very unsettling living with them.

One day my mom took me shopping at a mall in Las Vegas called Fashion Show. They had all the finest stores like Neimans, Dillards, and Saks Fifth Avenue – to name a few. She insisted I get whatever I wanted. I noticed her checking her watch. It made me suspicious, but I convinced myself that she was trying to be nice and I should give her a chance.

We loaded the car with our purchases and headed home. I was in my room putting my things away when the phone rang. She hollered to me that we needed to go to the ranch where Dandy was. I told her it was too hot as the temperature was in excess of 110 degrees. She ordered me into the car. As we arrived I noticed a truck with a horse trailer backing in. Perhaps a new horse was arriving? I couldn't have been more wrong.

The man exited his truck and approached my mother with a check. She had sold Dandy! I hadn't even been told she was up for sale. Dandy had been my everything for almost three years. I spent any free time I had with her. I poured my heart and soul out to her. My world was rocked to the core. I could barely breathe. I felt like I had the wind knocked out of me. This was my worst nightmare. This couldn't be real. I had maintained my end of our bargain. I kept my grades up and I never tried any drugs. Why was this happening?

They struggled to get Dandy into the trailer. She had never been trailered alone. She whinnied for me. I could feel her terror. I tried telling the man that she needed a trailer buddy. He refused to listen as he manhandled her into the trailer. Yet again, I was not listened to. I started crying hysterically; I could no longer watch it play out.

I am sorry my sweet girl, I loved you so much. Honestly, I still haven't healed from the grief of losing her.

As I started walking towards home, I saw my friend Kenny out in the desert with his falcon. Over the years I'd gotten to know my neighbor Kenny, who was around 18 years old, as I saw him on my way to and from visiting Dandy. Often high, Kenny was a mellow guy, an older brother type influence, who seemed to care about me and Tracy – something one notices with the lack of nurturing we received while children. As Kenny saw me walking that day, he noticed me crying and asked what happened. I told him what my mother had done. That moment Kenny lit up a joint and handed it to me. I had maintained my end of the bargain up until that day. Now all bets were OFF. I hated her for what she had done. I hated that I couldn't do anything about it.

I continued home after smoking the joint with Kenny. I was so angry at my parents for not preparing me for what had just gone down. My mom returned from the ranch and told me to get into the car again. She then drove to Sam's Town Casino with the check for Dandy. She headed directly to the cashier's cage, cashed the check, and bought several racks of silver dollars with the money she made from the sale. She then proceeded to put every last bit of it into the slot machines. Poof. Gone. She lost all of it. Dandy meant nothing to her, just money so she could gamble.

I was able to visit Dandy once after her sale. Her deep bay coat was bleached out from sun exposure. She had not been taken care of like I had cared for her. Dandy seemed distant and sad when I saw her. I never went back. I couldn't bear to see her again. I later learned she broke her neck while being trailered alone to Utah. What a tragic waste of such a magnificent creature.

I attended middle school in Vegas. I quickly fell in with the wrong crowd. I partied every weekend. My parents never noticed as they were consumed with their own problems. High school rolled around and things at home were not improving. After I turned 14 I bought myself a plane ticket to Wisconsin using my birthday money. I called my grandma from Denver and told her she needed to head to Madison to pick me up. I had left a note for my parents explaining my whereabouts. They did not come to retrieve me, in fact my sister followed behind a few months later.

Each summer I would return to Vegas to see my parents. Seeing them drinking themselves into a stupor every night reminded me of why I left in the first place. Every year I chose to return to Wisconsin in the fall. The dynamics of our family left little hope that we would ever be like the Norman Rockwell family I always dreamed of.

My mom heard about a back to school fashion show looking for models for an upcoming promotion at the Fashion Show mall. They were proud to announce that Top Model Twiggy would be assisting in choosing the models. I was super excited to be a part of the event. My mother bought me a beautiful suit to wear. My hair and makeup were flawless. I felt like it was my turn to dazzle. I took my spot on the catwalk. I had my head held high with a confident smile. I felt stunning!!

Twiggy waved me off the catwalk to come to her. I nervously approached her, feeling slightly nauseous, but not letting on. I smiled politely and listened as she told me I was a beautiful girl, but I had to lose my chubby cheeks. I managed to smile at her, but it was like someone knocked the wind right out of me. My heart sank immediately. I left Twiggy at the table, fighting back tears as I walked over to my mother. She couldn't wait to hear what Twiggy had said to me. When I told her what Twiggy had said, she told me not to worry about it. She promised that she would fix it. I wasn't sure what she meant by that, but I quickly found out.

The next day Mom drove me to a diet clinic. She forced me to go on their diet that would put my body into a fat burning mode called ketosis. It required me to get shots of B6 daily except Fridays when they shot me full of B12 to get me through the weekend. After a few weeks I collapsed in the clinic when they did a blood draw. My blood pressure dropped so low the clinic called an ambulance. I was one of their younger clients. They refused to treat me afterwards. I was grateful for that. However, this was when I began to hate my body, developed the feeling of never being good enough, and started struggling with an eating disorder. I started binging/purging and using laxatives to try and lose weight. Then I discovered speed. I could stay up for days at a time. All the other models were using it, and I found it erased my appetite. I used speed throughout high school. I developed a psychological condition known as body dysmorphia. I hated everything about my body.

Throughout high school I lived at Grandma's farm. I had been enrolled in junior and senior courses because I was an AT (academically talented) student in Vegas. I was always bored in school. In Wisconsin they had study halls which I found to be a massive waste of time. I often passed notes to friends and learned of weekend parties that were being organized. Since I looked older I was able to carry out liquor because none of the locals knew who I was. I was invited to the parties for this reason alone. Weekend road trips out in the country became my normal routine. To be completely honest I don't remember much from that time in my life. I was left to my own devices without much interference from my grandma who remained clueless of what we were doing. She trusted me and I was smart enough not to get into any major trouble. I loved my grandma deeply, but not myself.

I was set to graduate at midterm. Due to a virus I was unable to participate in Phy Ed. I had a doctor's excuse but the Phy Ed instructor demanded I stay another nine weeks to get the required quarter of a credit to graduate. Infuriated, I marched myself down to the library and took the GED tests. I passed all of them in the 90th percentile. I then threw it on my counselor's desk the following day and quit school. My counselor begged me to reconsider, but I refused.

Back in Vegas, my mother lined up a job for me at the nightclub where she was a bookkeeper. Tramps was the hot spot for businessmen lunches. Cecil, the manager, was known for hiring some of the most beautiful waitresses in town. I was a hostess. I enjoyed my job greeting people and making sure they enjoyed themselves while at Tramps. Men were always flirting with me. I took it all in stride. Everyone was so nice to me. One day my mother called me into her office. One of the regulars had requested that I join him in selecting the color for his new Porsche. She told me I should go with him. I was flattered and excited to get to ride in a Porsche.

The man picked me up from my parents house that afternoon and we headed to the dealership. He chose the color I liked. Of course I just agreed with whatever he said. My mom had made it clear to be polite and respectful, because he was a very influential man in Vegas. On the way home, we stopped at a casino for dinner. We got into the elevator for the restaurant but he wanted to make a stop at a room first.

I did not expect to be put into the compromising situation that unfolded next. He began to undress me and have his way with me. I was 17 years old at the time. I froze not knowing the best way to handle the situation. Although I was not a virgin, I was not very experienced. I felt disgusted and violated. He was well into his 40s and married. I was filled with shame and anger. When I returned home, my mom wanted to know all the details. I did not tell her what happened. Something told me that she knew exactly what went down.

Mom arranged another date for me with a man who was going to test drive a houseboat on Lake Mead. It was going to be a business purchase for entertaining clients. He had a captain and lunch waiting for us at the marina when we arrived. It was a massive and luxurious houseboat. It had all the bells and whistles imaginable. I felt like I was dreaming. I imagined what it would be like to be able to afford all of this! The captain took us out on Lake Mead while the man offered to take me "on a tour of the boat." Once again, I didn't expect the man to take me below deck and force himself onto me. I was alone and scared that if I didn't comply I wouldn't make it back to shore. The drive back to Vegas was very uncomfortable. An uneasy silence permeated his car. I was pissed to have been put into this situation by my mother once again. Upon my return home I informed her that I would no longer allow her to "hook me up" ever again!

I started to date other men. I dated a waiter from Tramps named Adrian. My mother hated him. That made it all the better. We dated briefly until I found out he had a longtime girlfriend. Betrayed by my mother and Adrian I finally decided to find another job.

I began working for a tour company that ran tours to Hoover Dam and flights through the Grand Canyon. I was hired for the sales department and was responsible for delivering commissions to the bell captains for booking our tours. I quickly won over the bell captains and sales increased. The owner John, 38, was very impressed. We started dating and I moved in with him. Anything to get out of my parent's house.

John was a very generous man. He took me shopping and bought me the best makeup and clothes. I had my hair highlighted and nails done. John wanted me to look my best so that his sales would continue to rise. I felt beautiful and appreciated. We took elaborate trips and ate at all the best restaurants. Life was good on the surface but things started to go downhill very quickly.

John liked to drink and he loved cocaine. From morning until night he was jacked up on coke. Weird things started happening. One night after we had been up for days, I felt like a shadow was standing over me while we were in bed. I chalked it up to lack of sleep, but the next morning when I woke up, my purse was gone. John figured I had left it at the office, but I knew I hadn't. Women don't leave their purses just anywhere.

At least I didn't. We arrived at the office in search of my purse. It was nowhere to be found. I was upset because now I would need to get a new driver's license and social security card just to do my job.

I was answering calls in the office when someone entered. As I looked up from my desk I saw something coming towards me. It was a stream of mace and the woman behind the can was John's ex-girlfriend Teresa. My eyes started burning and I screamed in pain as I ran down the hall to the bathroom to rinse my face. Teresa fled the scene. John raced in the bathroom to help me. I rinsed my eyes out thoroughly and then John drove me home to rest. I wanted her arrested but John wouldn't let me call the police. We left my car at the office because I couldn't see well enough to drive it home.

Upon our return to the office the next day I discovered my car's windshield had been shattered. A brand new Audi 80 that John had given me to use as a sales vehicle. WTH? It turned out he owed his dealer some money and the dealer was upset. My safety became an issue. John became extremely paranoid and began using tons of cocaine to stay up to drink and gamble. He would become abusive and violent if challenged. He attacked me several times because I voiced an opinion about something that didn't fully align with his. I became scared of him and then became depressed.

I went to a doctor because of severe headaches. He put me on a new drug called Prozac. I started to focus on a shotgun in the corner of our bedroom. I would fantasize about killing John the next time he attacked me. I returned for a follow up and mentioned it to my doctor. The Prozac was immediately stopped. However John's craziness continued.

One night I awoke to him coming up from the bottom of the bed under the sheets with a flashlight. He was poking and prodding my naked body. I kicked him right in the face. He totally freaked me out. I'd had enough and I started making my exit plan.

I had no money and if I left him I would lose not only my home but also my car and my job. I was screwed. We fought when he had too much to drink and would become belligerent. I taunted him and didn't care when he'd punch me in the face. I could never keep my mouth shut. Apparently I was too stupid to be afraid.

One night during a fight I went to use the toilet. John followed me into the bathroom, screaming at me while I was in there. As I finished my business and was standing up he quickly headbutted me in the face. As I fell to the ground, blood from my nose splattered everywhere. I was in disbelief. As he was screaming at me his teeth flew out of his mouth. I was shocked by what happened, but more shocked because I never knew he had false teeth! Who gets gapped tooth dentures?! What else didn't I know about him? He was ashamed of what he had done and immediately apologized. I didn't care. I had to find somewhere to go, but I was going to bide my time.

A few weeks went by and John had another meltdown and charged at me, rolling his ankle in the step-down living room. I moved out of the way as he charged me and he ended up falling flat on his face. I left him lying there in agony and went to my parents. He was getting crazier each time and I really thought he might kill me someday. I knew it was over; even if I had to return to my parents again, it wouldn't be for ever.

A few hours after I left him on the floor he called me, begging me to take him to the hospital. His ankle was so swollen that he couldn't drive his Porsche because it was a stick shift and he didn't want to call an ambulance. My mother told me to go and help him. She was sure he was sorry. I ended up taking him to the hospital. He apologized profusely and once again I forgave him. However, I was determined to have a place to go to when he was healed.

We managed to get along during his recovery. We took a trip to Jamaica and visited the Grand Cayman Islands while on a cruise. I no longer cared about him. I knew it was over. His coke habit made him into a person I wanted nothing to do with. I am not saying that I didn't partake in the partying, I did, but I saw the effects of longtime usage and it terrified me. We finally separated. His lawyer gave me a check for $5,000 to start my life over. I was grateful to have it.

I got myself a little Nissan Pulsar. A friend of mine was a salesman at a dealership and helped me to get my credit established. I began job hunting. I was hired at the Golden Nugget as a 24 Karat Club Hostess. I was paid to help high rollers enjoy their visit at the Nugget. We could issue room, food, or beverage comps. We could also arrange for limo transfers or flight arrangements. We would host elaborate parties based on the season or time of year. I was paid to be friendly and to help them have a good time. It was a great job.

There I met Jim. A retired air traffic controller, a man about the same age as my father. We started to have breakfast together after our late night shifts. We became close friends. Jim was a very sweet and caring gentleman. He fell in love with me, designed a beautiful ring, and proposed on the Fourth of July while we were visiting my grandma's farm. I was definitely caught off guard by his proposal. I said yes, but was immediately struck with the feeling that it was wrong. We returned to Vegas where I met his daughter and grandchildren. I realized that I wasn't ready to be a grandma or stepmother at age 21. I promptly returned his ring and moved back home, once again. I had no idea what the heck I wanted in my life. All

I had no idea what the heck I wanted in my life. All I had ever wanted was a family that loved me. I realized I was no good at relationships. I was tired of being hurt.

I had ever wanted was a family that loved me. I realized I was no good at relationships. I was tired of being hurt. I struggled with sadness for hurting Jim. It was never my intention, but it happened nonetheless.

I tried dating people after John, but it never went anywhere. One night I was returning home from work at the Nugget and it had started to rain. It was around 4 am when I went to sleep. I was jolted from sleep by the sounds of my grandma Helen screaming from down the hall. I sat up and my feet were submerged in about five inches of water. I ran down the hall to check on her. My dog Max, an 85-pound brindle boxer, was panicking because he hated the water. As I entered her room, her TV stand tipped over and launched her TV into the water. Luckily there was no power or we probably would have been electrocuted.

My parents were on their way home from New York where they'd been at a Yankees Old-Timers' game. I was supposed to have picked them up at the airport that morning. My alarm clock didn't go off because the power was out. Our entire cul-de-sac was under water. There were cars floating, slamming into one another. A neighbor said there were paramedics at the entrance of our street. They refused to enter the flood water to get my grandma out of the house. I needed to get her to them so I placed her on a pool raft and grabbed her catheter bag and Max and I pushed her towards the EMTs up the street. There were scorpions and cactus pieces floating in the water. Max was terrified and I had to keep my hand on his collar so he wouldn't drown.

My parents arrived in a taxi cab as Grandma was being tended to in the ambulance. They were shocked to return to their home under water. John had heard about the flooding from someone and showed up to help. A neighbor handed him a sledgehammer and both of them worked to break holes in the cinder block walls in our backyards to get the water back into the flood channel. John was high on coke, of course, but I was grateful for his help.

My parents and I spent the next several months redoing everything in the house. All carpeting and walls had to be removed and replaced. I lost all my shoes and purses that had been stored in the closets. Most of our photo albums were lost in the flood. Grandma Helen was transferred to a nursing home during the home repairs. Unfortunately she died there. She was in such a weakened state due to her poor health that she passed shortly after being admitted to the nursing home. There was no service for her. My mom said that's what she wanted since most of her friends passed or were living on the east coast.

I dove into my work. I picked up extra hours whenever possible. I helped my parents with the flood restoration. It was a great distraction for me for a while, but being with them was very difficult. Their drinking often resulted in loud screaming matches. My mom was always trying to find money to gamble.

She was always chasing a win to cover her recent losses. My father never called her out about her gambling. He acted like he was clueless about how bad she had gotten. Instead he expressed his hate for her by drowning himself in scotch every night. I usually hung out with friends after work to get away from their drama.

I wondered if I would ever find love. I hated living with my parents. I spent a lot of time alone in my room contemplating life. I began drinking more heavily. I prayed to God to bring me someone who would love me and not hurt me.

One night my girlfriends convinced me to come over and hang out with them at their apartment. We made daiquiris and hung out at the community pool and hot tub. Some new neighbors came over and introduced themselves. As it turned out, they were both metro policemen. We partied into the night and I went home with one of them. I don't remember much of anything afterwards, but, as luck would have it, I ended up pregnant.

My mother threw a fit and demanded I get an abortion. She threatened to put me out in the streets if I didn't. It went against what I believed in, but I didn't know what else to do. I was a mess. My mother confided in me that she had given up a baby for adoption and that she never wanted me to endure that pain. I believed her and, besides, I couldn't even take care of myself at the time.

Major depression took over my world following the abortion. I hated everything about myself. I questioned God about why nothing ever worked out for me. Why was I so unlovable? What was the point of life anyway? I needed to understand. I begged for clarification from God. Was love even possible for me?

I stayed home for months, only leaving the house for work. I would come home, drink, and sleep. I avoided my friends. I began drinking every night while home with the folks. Despite my loathing for them and telling myself I never wanted to be like them, I was emulating them. It was the only way I could tolerate living with them.

One night my friend Bobbie reached out. She was at the casino playing nickels and she met someone she thought I might like. Charles was a nice looking, clean cut man, dressed in khaki shorts and a polo shirt. He had a huge smile, a crazy sense of humor, and the ability to make me laugh – something I desperately needed at the time. We talked and drank throughout the night. I dropped him off at his mother's house the next morning.

Charles seemed nice, especially compared to other guys I'd been spending time with. He called me later that day and invited me to dinner. He wanted to make the most of his time in Vegas. We had a wonderful evening playing the slots and dancing in the lounge. I was finally out of my funk and able to enjoy life again. He was funny and didn't seem to have a care in the world. I invited him over to my parents' house for dinner. My mom told me she had a job interview that afternoon. I had him come over while she was gone so that we could have some privacy. Things got a little passionate and the next thing I know my mom barged in screaming for us to leave. Embarrassed and angered by her reaction, I gathered up my things and my dog and we checked into a motel for the evening. It was a dump, but we made due. I found a weekly apartment for us to stay at that was cheaper than the motel. We joked about getting married and how Mom would freak out. After many rum and cokes I decided: why not?! So we did. I would later regret that decision.

The first night in the apartment someone entered our room with a master key. Max alerted us to the intruder. Charles jumped out of bed and chased the man. He returned covered in blood. I asked if he was ok. He said "Yep, but the other guy didn't fare so well." Charles had grabbed a can of dog food as he ran out after the man. He put the can into a sock and used it as a weapon. WTH? I asked him where he came up with that idea and he calmly replied, "in prison." OMG, what have I gotten myself into? It wouldn't be long before I found out...

My grandma called and told me she was not feeling well. I had a terrible feeling, because she was a very strong woman. I decided we would go to Wisconsin to help her out.

Grandma was not well when we arrived. I immediately took her to the local hospital. They admitted her overnight.

They ran a bunch of tests and sent her home. They told her to collect a stool sample. She swore her stool was dark from eating beets. The next morning Charles and I were awakened with her screams from the bathroom. She was alarmed by the amount of blackness in her stool and the horrid aroma. I quickly called the hospital. We were ordered to get her to a hospital in Madison ASAP. After admitting her they discovered her aortic valve was leaking badly. She would need emergency surgery for a new valve. They cautioned us that at her age, however, it might be tricky.

I contacted my mom and told her about Grandma's situation. Mom wanted to be with her but didn't have any money for the flight. I offered to pay for her flight even though she and I were not getting along. I felt that she should be with her mother during this time. I called the airlines and made arrangements for her to come. It turned out to be a huge mistake.

I picked her up at the airport and offered to take her straight to the hospital. She wanted to be taken to the farm to pick up Grandma's car and then drive herself. Charles took my car and left to "go look for a job." Mom and I stayed as we were going to head into Madison later.

Once Charles left she started questioning me about him. I told her that I didn't want to talk about him. I was afraid she would call the cops and all hell would break loose. I reminded her that she was here to be with her mother during this time, not to start things back up with me. She began rifling through Grandma's desk. Then she began going through everything in the house. It really infuriated me. Finally, shit hit the fan between us. I reminded her that she was only here because Grandma might not survive the surgery. I wouldn't allow her to rummage through Grandma's things anymore. After a huge screaming match she jumped into Grandma's car and sped off. My head was pounding. She had a way of triggering me like no one else. Infuriated, I decided to take a hot bath and try to relax.

I had no sooner gotten into the tub when Charles burst into the bathroom. He was back from wherever he had been. He sat down on the toilet. I was telling him about what happened with my mom. As he was ripping off the toilet paper, the lattice strip the holder was attached to broke off. I said, "Great, you're gonna have to fix that!" In an instant, Charles launched off the toilet with the lattice strip in his hand and started hitting me in the bathtub with it – the staples from the lattice strips piercing my bare skin. I jumped out of the tub and ran outside to get away from him. He quickly followed behind. As I ran around a large bush in the yard, Max grabbed Charles' leg, pulling him to the ground, allowing me time to get inside. I locked the door behind me, leaving Charles outside. I grabbed a phone and a .22 rifle. I wasn't sure if it was even loaded but I held it pointed at his head through the patio door.

I phoned my friend Joe to come help me. Joe and his wife Ellie arrived within minutes from their farm. I handed the gun to Joe after he came inside the house. He told Charles to leave the property immediately to let things cool off. Ellie tended to me in the kitchen. Unbeknownst to me, Joe discreetly placed the rifle under a blanket on the couch in the back porch. Joe and Ellie left and I headed upstairs with a terrible migraine to lie down.

My mother returned while I was sleeping upstairs. She called the police because she found the gun hidden under the blanket on the couch that she had been sleeping on. She claimed it was intended as a threat by me and she feared for her safety. They questioned me about why the gun was there. I told them that Joe had put it there, careful not to elaborate about Charles and the fight. The cops questioned my mom about how much she had to drink. They could clearly smell it on her. Nothing else was done. They left and took the gun down to Joe's house for safekeeping. As they were leaving Charles was returning. They passed each other on the gravel road. Charles freaked out! He demanded that I immediately pack our things and off we went.

We had no destination in mind, but he thought he would be able to make some money if we headed to Florida. He was furious that my mother had called the cops. I tried calming him down but he went ballistic on me. He started to beat me with his fist while he was driving. He was swerving all over the road, Max was standing in the back of my CRX trying desperately to get his footing. I ordered him to stop and it made him angrier. He pounded on me more. I couldn't breathe because he had literally knocked the wind out of me. We drove into Chicago heading south towards Florida. He wanted to score some weed. I called a friend of mine to get some. We checked into a motel. He made me leave Max with him so he knew I would return. I went to my friend's and quickly returned with some weed to calm him down.

Over the next few weeks, we made our way to Florida using my credit cards and the Traveler's Checks his mother had given him. Turns out they were stolen and the keys were master sets for RV campers. I learned that he came from a long line of con artists. His abuse on me continued for weeks. He would leave me at the motel while he went looking for ways to make some money. One day he returned with a gun. He thought it would be funny to hold it near my head when we had sex. Now after being raped and beaten, I was determined to get away from him. We had maxed out my credit cards. He finally made a dire mistake when he abandoned me and my dog in a motel where we were later evicted.

That night I called his mother from a payphone in the lobby. I told her what had happened and how he had stolen my car. She insisted that I not to do anything to Charles or she would go after my family. I told her to go to hell. Max and I sat on the curb outside the motel for hours. Charles finally returned at 3 am. Luckily, the front desk clerk had overheard me talking to his mother and called the police. They arrived and immediately took him into custody to be extradited back to California. He was wanted by the state of California for leaving the state and failure to report. There was just enough gas in my car to make it into Georgia. Once there, I sold what jewelry I had at a pawn shop and headed back to Wisconsin. I had to know what happened to my grandma.

No one was at the farm when I returned. My mom listed and sold her 113-acre farm for a measly $72,000. She then took grandma back to Nevada. With nowhere else to go, I stayed at Joe and Ellie's because I couldn't find a place that would allow Max. I worked daily on Joe's dairy farm for three weeks. I helped him with milking chores and feeding the animals. We also cut and stored firewood for the winter. I was safe at Joe's but absolutely was not up to the intense manual labor that comes with farming. I looked up an old friend, Jerome, and he found somewhere Max and I could crash.

Jerome's friend Gale welcomed me and Max. We became fast friends. Gale loved animals and Max loved him. It was a good sign. Finally I had a physical address and had my mail forwarded. I finally saw the damage from running with Charles. In less than three months my credit cards maxed out at over $17,000. I didn't know what to do. I took several part time bartending jobs. I thought I might have to declare bankruptcy. Gale drove me into Madison to speak with an attorney. The attorney advised me against declaring bankruptcy, because I was involved in a lawsuit along with my parents regarding their home flooding and I may receive a monetary settlement. We left the attorneys and headed home, stopping at the Sandbar Sports Arena for a drink to lighten the mood.

An Unexpected Change

The Sports Arena, in Arena, Wisconsin, was formerly a commercial chicken coop. It was huge. It had indoor horseshoe pits and volleyball courts. It was brimming with activity. As we sat down, Dave, the owner, took our drink order. I commented about what a cool place it was and inquired if they were hiring. Dave hired me on the spot. We stayed there and drank for hours. I had a great time. The next morning, fuzzy headed, I asked Gale if I had really gotten the job. He assured me that Dave was serious and I was supposed to work that night.

I curled my hair, put on some makeup, and headed to the Sports Arena. I wanted to make a good impression. I met Dave and he quickly got me acclimated to the bar. The first two men I waited on asked me where I came from. I told them I was from Vegas. They asked if I was a showgirl or dancer and wanted to know how I ended up in Arena. I told them my father retired from baseball and moved us to Vegas when I was a child. Their tone excitedly changed, inquiring who my father was. It turned out one of the men, Gene Brabender, was roommates with my father when they played together for the Orioles. Such a small world! I couldn't believe it. I called my dad and handed the phone to Gene. They talked briefly. Gene and Jerry were regular customers. They welcomed me into their small town. I worked the weekend and was asked to come in for Volleyball night on Monday. A few of the customers requested me as the bartender for the evening. Dave agreed to bring me in, but they would have to make it worthwhile and stay for drinks after the volleyball session.

My life was about to change forever. I wasn't looking for another man. I was still trying to figure out how to terminate my marriage to Charles. While I was with Charles I had prayed to God repeatedly to rescue me from the relationship. I prayed for a hero. I prayed constantly while I was in the midst of his abuse. That night God answered my prayers – big time!

In walked Bryon. I was 24 and he was 35. He was there to fill in for someone for co-ed volleyball. His wife had left him only five days earlier, when she ran off with the horse trainer. He was devastated and his friends were consoling him. Everyone drank until closing. Randy, one of Bryon's friends, invited me back to Bryon's house for a drink. After much encouragement I followed them to Bryon's. When we got to his house we all headed directly into his basement bar. The bar was beautifully made with rocks from the property and it was fully stocked. Everyone was having a great time. Randy and his friend left Bryon's around 4 am. Bryon and I talked until the sun rose. We had an undeniable connection. And though neither of us were looking for another relationship, God had other plans for us.

That night I became sick from drinking too much. Bryon helped hold my hair out of the toilet. I told him I wanted to take a shower. He stood clothed in the shower while I cleaned up. I was so ashamed, but he didn't seem to care. He was a perfect gentleman. He even washed my clothes for me and gave me something to wear. He never attempted to take advantage of me in my drunken condition. I was grateful that he seemed to be a good guy for a change. This was a clear nudge from God, the universe, or whatever you care to call it. Bryon would be my answered prayer. Bryon became the hero I always needed in my life.

We laid down fully clothed to rest for a bit. Suddenly we were awoken to his wife slamming the bedroom door. She had stopped in to feed her horses and found us sleeping. He ran after her, and told me to stay put. Ever the stubborn one, I quickly "beat feet" and headed home.

Bryon showed up at the Sports Arena later that night while I was working. I apologized profusely for getting sick and causing him any issues in possibly rekindling his marriage. He assured me that his marriage was over. I informed him I needed to deal with getting my marriage annulled. I didn't want to be in a relationship and neither did he. The attraction between us was strong. Here I go again, falling in love, dammit.

While we were ecstatic to be together, his son was not. Bryon Jr. wasn't into his dad having a new girlfriend. He was just turning 14 – a tough age for kids anyway. He thought I was a big mouthed blonde and he wasn't going to make it easy for me. He pulled all sorts of crap to try to run me off. Like telling me that his dad would never marry me, I was just a distraction, etc. When I would talk to Bryon about Junior's disrespect, he would say we were like brother and sister, and he wouldn't take any action to correct the problem. Finally, after over a year together I'd had enough. I told them I was leaving and they could help pack and move my things into storage. They could have each other. Max and I returned to Vegas.

I stayed with my girlfriend Bobbie for three weeks. Bryon and I talked daily. We tried to resolve things long distance, but it went nowhere. We both wanted to work it out. We both loved each other. We were very clear on that. He wanted me to return to Wisconsin. He flew out to Vegas, got us a suite at the MGM Grand, and then drove me and Max back to Arena. Junior never spoke nasty or disrespectfully to me again. I knew I was where I was meant to be. I knew Bryon loved me and I knew I loved him immensely. God was answering my prayers for a family.

We got engaged about two years later when I was eight months pregnant with Brody. Bryon proposed to me while we were fishing on the Chippewa Flowage. We had intended to spend the weekend fishing and camping on an island. He navigated the boat into a secluded cove and he slipped the ring on my finger. I was ecstatic! I couldn't wait to tell our friends and family. We cut our camping trip short and returned home. Our friends, Vern and Evy, had planned a couples baby shower for us the following weekend. Upon my return we contacted a justice of the peace and changed the party from baby shower to wedding reception. I called my parents expecting them to be overjoyed, but they were less than responsive. Even though we offered to pay for their tickets, they declined to attend. They never even sent a wedding gift. Regardless, our wedding day was perfect.

Our friends graciously allowed us to use their beautiful estate for our wedding. We were married on their flagstone patio next to a large, beautiful fountain. There was a gorgeous view of the countryside. The justice of the peace provided the music, *The Rose* by Bette Midler, on a boombox. I was an emotional and very pregnant bride, fighting back tears through the whole song. My dream was coming true! I finally found my prince! After the wedding the host's brother flew his small plane over the reception dumping confetti in celebration. It missed us by a mile, but to me it was magical. We celebrated around a large bonfire into the night. Everyone had brought a dish to pass. His brother Tod supplied us with 46 pounds of smoked salmon that he'd caught in Alaska. It was quickly devoured by our guests. We supplied all the beverages which was the biggest expense of our wedding. Bryon's first mother-in-law, Edna, made us a gorgeous three tiered wedding cake. She had made all three of Bryon's wedding cakes! Everything went perfectly. My dreams were all coming true. My son's birth would turn out to be my next blessing.

Blessed with Birth

Brody was born a month later. My water broke at home. He was an easy delivery, It was only four hours of labor pains. He was perfect – smart, beautiful, and happy! I loved being a mother. My dream came true, I had a son! Bryon would sit up with me during the night when I breastfed. I would look at this baby with such love and awe. Yet something wasn't right with me. I couldn't stop crying. I thought it was because I was a new mother, but it was more than that. I had developed postpartum depression. I was put on antidepressants. I had to quit breastfeeding, and I quickly went back to drinking. We enjoyed the next year being parents to Brody.

Bryon's 40th birthday came around. I threw him a surprise party at a local tavern. I invited all of his family and friends. I had a special cake made and the rest of the food was catered. Friends of his asked how he enjoyed being a dad again. He mentioned that we were thinking of having another child. His mother, Lila, quickly ran into the restroom, returning with a handful of condoms that she jammed into the front pocket of his jeans in view of the whole party. Little did we know at the time but I was already pregnant. Jake was born the following August.

Jake's birth was awful. I spent over eight hours in labor. He was a large baby. There were a lot of births on the same day he was born. They struggled to find a doctor to deliver him. Finally they caught one heading into the clinic and rushed her in to help me. My cervix was twisted so I had a bunch of pillows placed under me to get the baby off the cervix so it could be untwisted. Once that was completed he was delivered instantly, tearing my nether region to shreds. Afterwards, I swore it was the last baby.

I left the hospital later the same day to return home to Brody. I should've stayed in the hospital. I was exhausted. The next day Lila came to see the new baby. As we were talking in my kitchen I got a weird sensation between my legs. I rushed down the hall to the bathroom. As I went to sit on the toilet a large blood clot the size of a softball fell into my panties. Panicked, I called out to Lila, as she was the only one there. She came into the bathroom, saw the clot, and quickly ran for something to put it into. I composed myself and called the hospital to see if it was anything urgent. They assured me it was normal and to just throw it away.

Jake was a very quiet baby. Often he wouldn't wake to feed. I would wake up soaking wet with breast milk. Panicking that something was wrong I would run to Jake to wake him to eat. I worried constantly. I knew something wasn't quite right with him. He was delayed in reaching milestones. He never really babbled. He would entertain himself by watching his hands. He would spend hours lining up Hot Wheel cars and just stare at them. In the bath he was very content just spinning shampoo bottles in their holder. Finally, at 17 months, we found out he might be Autistic.

Knowing nothing about Autism Spectrum Disorder, I dove into the internet reading everything I could. I enrolled him into The Wisconsin Early Autism Program. He had intensive therapy for eight hours every day. Our house was a revolving door of therapists. Jake received 40 hours of therapy a week for the next three years. Anything to give him a chance at having a normal life. We met a special therapist named Joyce who became like part of our family. She had a background in child development. Jake responded well to her approach and definitely her patience with him. I hired her exclusively to be his full time therapist. She became a close friend of mine during the 15 years that she was with us.

Secretly I was riddled with guilt and shame. I blamed myself for his condition. I thought he was Autistic because I had consumed alcohol before realizing I was pregnant. I hated myself. The antidepressants didn't seem to help with my depression, but they were great for killing my sex drive and putting on weight. I wasn't sleeping. I was anxious all the time about Jake.

Brody started school. Jake was busy with therapists. I was overwhelmed with guilt and feared for his future. I worried about him being unable to take care of himself. I feared that I would never be able to achieve my dreams of traveling. I felt as though some of my freedoms were diminishing as Jake's needs would have to come first. I had to let go of the dreams I had for Jake's future. It was a type of grieving process. My overthinking brain was constantly searching for possible solutions for his future.

I continued to learn everything I could about Autism. I wanted to give Jake every chance at leading a normal, fulfilling life. I needed to find a way that he could have a normal future. I became his advocate, mentor, and motivator. I knew God brought Jake into our world for a special reason. No matter how hard it might be, I knew we would be okay. I felt that deep within my heart. There was still a sense of grief that I didn't expect with Jake's diagnosis. I had to allow myself to mourn the life I had imagined for him. I feared that I would never be able to achieve my dreams of traveling, because Jake would never be able to live unsupervised.

It took me a while, but at some point I realized that Jake's disability was actually a gift. I had never been around anyone with Autism prior to this. I was eager to learn everything I could. As an empath I have always put myself in others' shoes. I wondered what it would be like to be like my son. I studied him to understand how he thinks. I started to notice the unique things about Jake like how he had a fantastic memory. He would line up 30 Hot Wheels cars in a row and knew the exact order of each car. Occasionally we would switch the order of a couple of the cars while he was distracted. Immediately he would catch it and quickly put them back where they belonged. During the first three plus years of his life he couldn't speak. We learned some sign language to help him have his needs met. We introduced PECS cards (Picture Exchange Communication System) to help him communicate with us. ABA (Applied Behavior Therapy) helped him to follow commands. Slowly he began making progress. I learned about different programs to help kids like Jake. When he was four he began to approximate words. He was enrolled in the early childhood program at school and filled the rest of his day with therapy at home with Joyce. This continued throughout his school career.

During this time I was also taking care of my aging grandmother. She was struggling with early dementia. I had to call her by 8 am daily or she would become upset. If it was after 8, she wouldn't answer the phone and I would have to run to her apartment to make sure she wasn't hurt or dead. It was difficult for me to please everyone. I was exhausted by being a caregiver and constantly worried about Grandma and Jake. Trying to make things work for everyone involved and being the perfect wife and mother was overwhelming.

I started having chest pain radiating in my sternum and then my left arm would go numb. I would begin to sweat profusely. A few times I was rushed to the hospital thinking I was dying only to be dismissed as having panic attacks. I was given lots of anxiety meds and discharged. This went on for two years. I began to question my sanity. I would experience terrible chest pain only to be told over and over again it was a panic attack – and that there was nothing wrong with me. But I knew something wasn't right. Yet again, I wasn't truly listened to. Bryon was growing weary as it all seemed like a ploy for attention. I languished in limbo while I was loaded on meds and booze.

My Life Changed Forever

On February 19, 2004, at age 35, I suffered a cardiac arrest. Both my children were home at the time. Jake was working with a therapist in his room. Brody was home with a nasty tooth infection. Bryon came in from the shop for lunch. He found me blue lipped and lifeless on the bathroom floor. He promptly called 911 and began CPR. The fire chief arrived with a defibrillator. Luckily he only lived a few miles from our home. He hooked up the defibrillator and it immediately delivered a shock. As it was preparing to deliver another shock, a faint pulse was detected. I was quickly loaded into the ambulance and taken to Sauk Prairie Hospital. When I came to in the ambulance I was completely blind. Vicky, an EMT, tried to calm me down as we raced to the hospital. I became somewhat combative, common with a brain injury. When we arrived at the hospital the doctors read the defib tape and sent me immediately to another hospital in Madison where an ICD (internal cardiac defibrillator) was implanted in my chest. I had gone without oxygen for an unknown period of time resulting in an anoxic brain injury. It basically destroyed my short-term memory.

As Arena's first volunteer EMTs to save a life with a defibrillator, they were honored by the state at a medical convention at the Kalahari Resort in Wisconsin Dells. Bryon and I gave our account of the events in front of a large audience of doctors and nurses. It was surreal. I struggled to believe everything that had happened. Was this a dream or more of a nightmare? It was yet to be determined.

I was a busy mom to two active boys. I was the sole caretaker for my aging grandmother. I had no help from my family. My parents didn't even visit during this time. My dad's health was poor. Years of smoking cigarettes and heavy drinking were catching up with him. My mother and I had a tumultuous relationship throughout my life. I had no one to confide in but my husband and clearly he had been traumatized by my cardiac arrest. My friends didn't come around. The people I thought would always be there for me disappeared. Depression took over my world. I began drinking

> *I was able to stay sober for about a year and a half. I always managed to sabotage myself with boredom or some lame excuse to pick up. I didn't like myself, much less love myself. Years of trauma and neglect by my family and people close to me left me angry and rebellious.*

heavily every day. Disgusted with myself, I voluntarily checked myself into rehab – 30 days of inpatient therapy. Alcohol had destroyed my family while I was growing up. I promised myself that I would never be like them. Yet, here I was trying to cope with life with rum and Diet Pepsi.

I was able to stay sober for about a year and a half. I always managed to sabotage myself with boredom or some lame excuse to pick up. I didn't like myself, much less love myself. Years of trauma and neglect by my family and people close to me left me angry and rebellious. Now with a brain injury it was difficult for me to create new memories. I stayed stuck, replaying the events from the past. Realizing that alcohol and pain went well together, I knew I was slowly killing myself yet I wanted to be numb.

My lifelong friend, Jim, came to visit from Illinois. We stopped at the local cheese store to buy some cheese curds. As I hurried into the store my foot caught the rug's edge and I fell to the ground. I ended up breaking my elbow and ankle, and spraining my wrist. They x-rayed my neck because I had neck issues as well. During the x-ray it was discovered that I had nodules throughout my lungs. A CT scan of my lungs then revealed a mass in my liver. I developed an autoimmune disease called Polymyalgia Rheumatica (PMR). The treatment is steroids, mainly Prednisone. I ballooned up to 300 pounds. I had a heart attack in my doctor's office and was rushed to Madison once again. I immediately had two stents placed in the arteries surrounding my heart.

Thankfully, a lovely nurse recommended cardiac rehab to help me regain strength. I was so moved by her compassion that I reluctantly agreed. At rehab, a joyful, exuberant nurse greeted me. I hated her instantly. She radiated joy. Who does that? Certainly not me – not then, anyway. I was fitted with a heart monitor and led into the exercise room. Immediately, I felt like I'd stepped into an old folks' home. What was I doing here? I don't belong here. I reluctantly started the treadmill, giving only half-hearted effort. An elderly man stepped onto the treadmill beside me, smiling politely. "Oh God, I'm in hell." The machine started, and suddenly grandpa was running flat out next to me. Meanwhile, I was beet red, sweating profusely, barely moving at one mile an hour. I knew something had to change, but I wasn't ready. I still didn't love myself. I languished for years, living in limbo. No goals, no plans – until life happened.

My father succumbed to COPD and pneumonia complications. My mother had him removed from the ventilator system on Super Bowl Sunday and he passed shortly after. A few months later my mother and grandmother moved to Wisconsin to be closer to me. Shortly after arriving in Wisconsin my beloved grandmother passed away. The following year, I found my mother dead 12 days before Christmas. I believe she finally decided to quit drinking and it caused her death. We were in the midst of finally having a mother daughter type relationship that I'd always dreamed of. We had made some progress, but it was cut short by her death. I spiraled out of control. I was sober before she died, but quickly picked up again and tried to drown myself consuming a handle of rum every three days.

Tracy's Tragedy

After my mom died in 2008, I gave Tracy the contents of her apartment. She was so grateful and happy for everything. Unfortunately, it didn't last. Tracy was a recovering meth addict and longtime alcoholic. She was a beautiful and brilliant woman who had succumbed to her demons. Tracy got some guy to bring an open back trailer to Wisconsin to pick up Mom's things. On their way back they lost several pieces of furniture off the truck. Unfortunately Tracy couldn't keep a place, and ended up putting all the furniture on a curb for free.

Years later, in 2016, I was called to the hospital as Tracy had been placed on life support when her organs began to shut down. As the only surviving family member I was called to sign the papers allowing them to remove her from life support. She would not be recovering this time. My sister was nine months and two days younger than me. We were like twins. She was all I had left of my immediate family. I felt empty and alone.

I flew to Mississippi and met a friend who drove me to Georgia. We entered her hospital room and noticed her restrained to the bed. She thrashed around and mumbled incoherently. She didn't even acknowledge my presence. Her brain was toxic from years of alcohol abuse. Her boyfriend approached me promising to never let her drink again once she was released. I explained to him that she would not be going home this time.

I signed the papers, the nurses let me say goodbye to her, and we left. She was removed from life support the next morning and they called me after she took her last breath. I handled her cremation arrangements and returned home to Wisconsin. A few weeks later her remains were delivered to my house.

My sister left behind twin teenage boys. It broke my heart that they would never see Tracy again. I didn't want that fate for my boys. I knew that I needed to make changes in my life. I would be the one to break the generational curse.

On August 29, 2019, my son drove me to the hospital to detox. I promised him that this would be the last time. I promised myself this was my last chance. I was in a very dark, lonely, isolated place and my health was terrible. I was emotionally, physically, and spiritually drained. I challenged God to help me or take me home. I knew I was powerless over my life. I wanted to join my family wherever they were. I wanted out, but God revealed to me that I was needed. When I surrendered my will to God I immediately felt lighter. I started to feel like I had worth. I felt God's love for me.

Taking Back Control of My Life

I found myself a therapist and began CBT (cognitive behavioral training) to deal with my PTSD and depression issues. I also got myself a psychiatrist who realized that I had a circadian rhythm disorder and prescribed a new medication for sleep. I was finally able to get the restorative sleep that had eluded me for years.

My therapist knew I was struggling with body dysmorphia and was very conscious of my huge weight gain. To improve my body image she recommended journaling and practicing gratitude each day. As I was journaling, my life would come to me in rhyme. I eventually published my poems and dedicated my first book to my medical team for helping me through my health issues over these past 20 years. I'm including some of these poems later in this book.

I quit smoking cigarettes after 36 years. I quit cold turkey after my doctors kept blaming all my health issues on smoking. I challenged them to find out the real cause after convincing myself that they weren't the problem. I kept a pack of cigs on the end table near my bed. I would look at it each day determined not to remove the cellophane wrapper and smoke one. It became a battle of wills. A year after quitting we had a large bonfire with some friends to celebrate the official end of my cigarette smoking days. I threw that pack of cigs into the flames to celebrate being cigarette free at last!

I began working out with a friend. I really needed someone to hold me accountable. I had muscle wasting due to years being sick and stuck in bed. We had to begin very slowly – first chair yoga and eventually worked our way up to Zumba type dancing. Struggling through injuries as a result of the long term Prednisone usage, I slowly took off 85 pounds over the next four years. Multiple injuries made it difficult to be consistent. Physical therapy became a regular event for me. Despite the seemingly constant setbacks, I was determined to continue. I was loving the changes I was seeing in myself.

I got a nutritionist. Actually she turned out to be Miss Happy from Cardiac therapy! We eventually became good friends. She is the one who encouraged me to publish my poetry books! Actually, she's the one who helped me love myself. Because of her I developed better eating habits. I also began using supplements to heal myself. I eventually got off a bucketful of medications. I am doing things holistically these days whenever possible. I am now able to work again. I help seniors and people with disabilities live independently in their homes. I love my clients. They have become like family to me.

Glory to God

These past 21 years since my cardiac arrest have helped me to understand the importance of helping others and the importance of giving others second chances. I have come to understand grief and resilience. I have learned that we must never give up on ourselves. We must be mindful that everyone is struggling with something. We all have a story.

My surrendering to God revealed my purpose. By being of service to others I found the happiness that eluded me for most of my life. I wake each day eager to see what God has planned for me today. I am mindful to remember to practice gratitude. I listen to a daily devotional each morning. I take things one day at a time and I give myself grace. On days that don't go my way I look for the lesson. I discovered that happiness is a choice. Instead of focusing on all the wrongs of this world, I make a conscious effort to look for the good in things.

20 years ago I was a woman without a purpose; it turned out my death was the new beginning that I needed.

20 years ago I was a woman without a purpose; it turned out my death was the new beginning that I needed.

During my Bible studies, I was told the story of Job. It was an "aha" moment – I finally understood what God wanted me to see. If you don't know the story, Job's life was full of struggle. He endured many trials from Satan, yet never lost his faith in God. I saw myself in Job. A man of means, he lost animals he treasured – sheep and cattle stripped from him. I knew how it felt to lose something I loved deeply, comparing it to the loss of my beloved Dandy. Job lost his family. Mine were gone as well. I felt abandoned after the deaths of my parents, grandmother, and sister. What struck me most was when, after losing everything, Satan cursed him with a horrific skin disease, covering him with abscesses and boils. The description is very similar to my own condition, Hidradenitis Suppurativa (HS). Even with everything thrown at him, Job's faith carried him through. I credit my faith for sustaining my life today. God has helped me endure incredibly difficult trials. I am alive to testify to God's love for each of us.

Why I Write Poems

I often write poems as a way to process my emotions. My brain is constantly working overtime. I analyze everything that happened throughout my day, week, month, year, etc. My brain rarely takes a break and I struggle constantly with getting rest. My sleep is disruptive and frustrating. I wake up thinking of upcoming commitments or solutions to something that troubled me earlier. Always thinking. I have to tell my brain to give these things to God. As a person who fears loss of control this is very challenging. I understand now, though, that God's ways are best for me. I have learned to love myself during this journey, so I give these worries to Him on a regular basis.

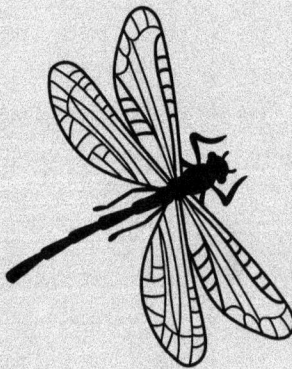

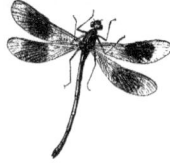

Just Take It

Why must life be so hard?
Why does love always break my heart?

Everything seems to end in pain.
I try so hard to change that it drives me insane.

I feel like a phony who will soon be discovered
I realize that no one really cares if I ever recover.

I act real confident; just like a pro.
Yet inside I'm unraveling I want you to know.

All my life I've been told to be strong.
To just take it; even though I did nothing wrong.

I hate that I've become this way.
I've tried everything else; now I chose to pray.

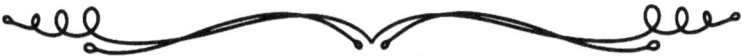

**Just because they are beautiful and
smiling doesn't mean they are happy...**

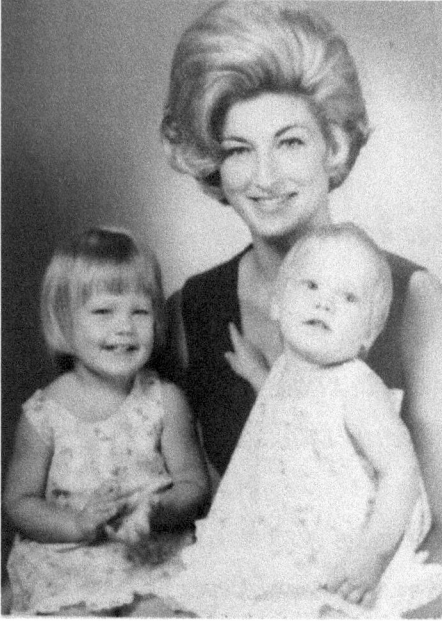

Dani, Mom, Tracy

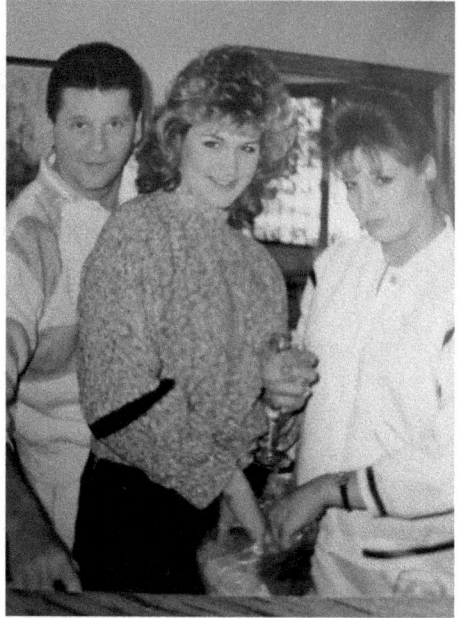

John, Dani, Tracy (at Christmas party)

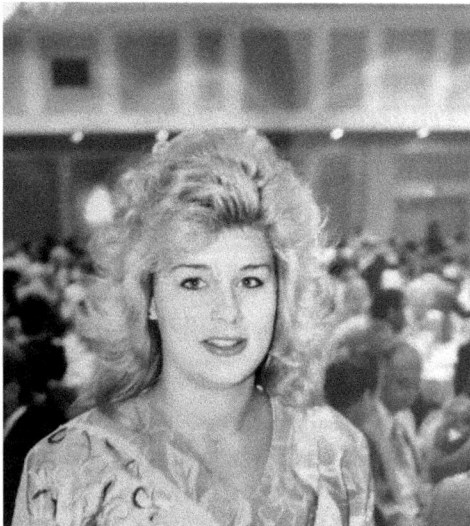

Dani at Dad's
induction into
Baltimore Orioles
Hall of Fame
1988

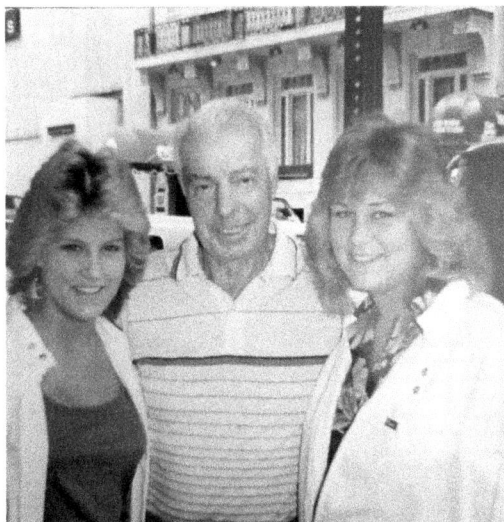

Tracy, Joe Dimaggio, Dani
at Dad's induction

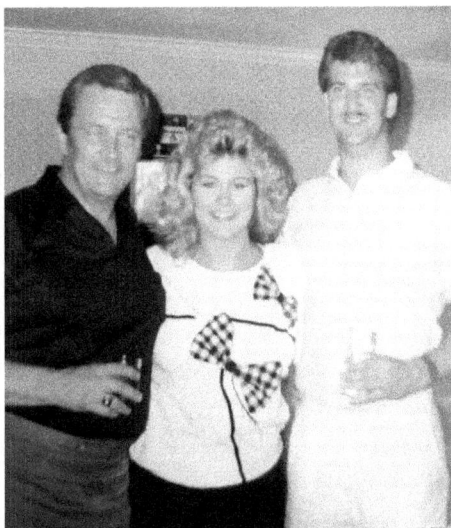

Dad, Dani, Steve (half brother)

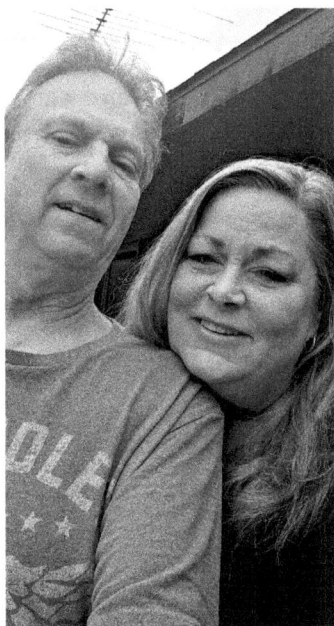

Bryon and Dani
Coming through it all together,
with my rock

Finding God & Seeing Miracles

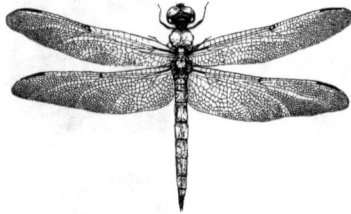

My faith has allowed me to renew my relationship with God. Raised Catholic, I walked away from the church for various reasons. I did not stop believing in God. Raised on my grandmother's farm I spent lots of time out in nature. I had 113 acres to get lost in. I studied the birds and creatures I encountered. I would imagine what it would be like to be them. I understood how each creature was a part of the forest and contributed a unique purpose. I noticed how the plants provided for the bugs, who provided for the animals, who provided for humans, etc. Everything had a purpose. They instinctively know their purpose. I never knew my purpose in life. I never thought I really mattered. I mean I am only one of millions of people, right? God showed me that I do matter.

On this journey of life I wanted to understand WHY. Why all of this? Why should I care? Why do I have to keep struggling over and over? I did not understand that I had become a victim of life. When I was complaining about this or that repeatedly I was actually allowing the universe to bring me more of that kind of thing into my life. Whining to the universe about how unfair things were for me just ensured that life would continue to give me more of what I was focusing on. Negative energy attracts more negative results. Once I understood this, I flipped the script. I no longer languished in the misery that I had allowed to take over my life previously. I focused instead on what I wanted my life to be like. I focused my energy on getting my health and strength back.

I had struggled for so long to find purpose in my life before I surrendered myself to God. I truly needed to find a reason to remain on the planet. I was so consumed with being a victim in my life. A victim of things that others had done to me. Whether it was ex-lovers, friends, or even well meaning doctors, I became their victim in my mind somehow. Hurt or betrayed for trusting family members, and others, who claimed to have cared about me. Resulting in me withdrawing from the world and suffering from isolation and loneliness. I had plenty of reasons for wanting to die, but my faith told me to hang on. When I surrendered, I was pulled from despair by God's love and understanding. He showed me how I mattered. He revealed my purpose to me that day. He has a purpose for each and every one of us.

God gifted me with an understanding that day. He showed me that I had gotten through everything throughout my life because of God's love for me. He asked me to give myself the love I so freely gave to others. These days I focus on staying in alignment with Him. There is nothing better in this world than when you are one with the universe. I am a divine child of God. You are too. I hope you take the time to explore and nourish your spiritual side. God opened my eyes and there's no looking back for me!

I started thanking God for everything in my life. My husband, my kids, a beautiful home, and especially for restoring my health. I was grateful that He was bringing the right people into my life. I wanted to please Him. I prayed for guidance and discernment. I prepared my heart to be open and receptive for whatever God brought to me.

I begged to learn His word. I struggled with reading the Bible. Having ADHD makes reading a challenge. I am easily distracted and find it difficult to understand names listed in the Bible. God remedied that struggle for me when he brought Andrea into my life. She is very educated in the teachings of the Bible. We began studying together at our weekly meetings. She began talking about Job and she told me of all his struggles throughout his life. I felt an instant connection when she spoke of his skin condition and the boils he endured.

My HS skin condition has caused me great stress since my adolescence. I would get these incredibly painful cysts that

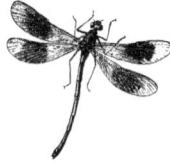

By God's Design

The beauty from God is all around.
Nothing is a mistake when a purpose can be found.

The trees are in their glory as they shed their leaves.
They have been created by God's design;
another reason to believe.

It amazes me that He thought enough to create the four seasons.
No detail was overlooked, everything had a reason.

He loves everything about us; for we were all designed
To be imperfect creatures; inspired by His mind.

He gave us emotions to help us understand.
What love and joy feels like, that was His plan.

Now I can share my love for others.
With God at the center we can unite with one another.

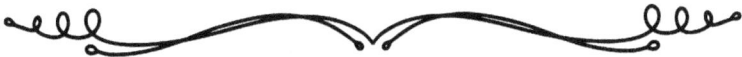

would often smell horrible. I was embarrassed and ashamed of this disorder because they would pop up in the most awful places and I would have to go in for them to be drained. I never dared to talk about them, fearing the judgment of these disgusting things. I related to Jobs' stories with struggles. I became excited to learn more about God's word. The more I learn the more I am able to see how it is still relevant in the world today! Now if I have a setback with my health or finances, I remember how much one can endure. I now look for the lessons in my struggles. What is it I could learn from the situation? Then I thank God for the blessings that I have today in my life.

Recently I believe God intervened on my behalf when I had a recurrence of PMR. I was feeling more tired and stiff than usual for a few days, then weeks, but I kept trying to push through it. Finally one morning I could barely make a fist or lift my arms above my shoulders. I had blood drawn to check my inflammation markers, and it became apparent that the PMR was back, requiring me to restart the Prednisone protocol. I was horrified to think I would be putting all the weight I'd lost back on and I would also be gaining the wonderful moon face back to my appearance. Bryon tried to cheer me up, but I was inconsolable. I was angry and in pain. I quickly started to go down the "poor me" path again. Why should I even bother to try and improve my life when these health problems continue to plague my life? Why should I put my faith in God when

He doesn't end my suffering? My brain sensed the message, "humble yourself before God." Then I remembered Job and all he endured in his life. I began pleading for God's mercy and Grace. I prayed that He would make a way for me without the use of steroids. I begged for forgiveness in not appreciating all the good in my life and promised to do better.

The next morning when I got out of bed I noticed that I wasn't as stiff as I had been. My wrists and hands didn't hurt as badly. I had waited to start the steroids until the morning, but here I was able to move without them. Could it really be that simple? I went about my appointments, I told myself I would wait a bit just to make sure I was improving. Noon came around for my meeting with my publisher. I realized my pain was much more manageable without the use of steroids. God had answered my prayers once again.

I am grateful for my relationship with God. Everyday I am in awe of His creations. I have seen him work miracles in my life. I look for glimmers every day. Nods from the universe. God in action. No small detail has been overlooked. God has thought of everything. You just have to be open and willing to see what He is trying to show you. Glimmers are gifts meant for those of us who are enlightened by His love. I used to believe I was insignificant; just another person on the planet. Now I know that God made each of us by his design with a specific purpose. I encourage you to discover your purpose and live the life that God always wanted for you.

Miracles

I don't know how many times God helped me through something, and I'm grateful for that.

The definition of a miracle according to Google: is a surprising and welcome event that is not explicable by natural or scientific law and is therefore considered to be a work of a divine agency.

I have been a witness to many miracles throughout my life. During these times I didn't realize the significance of these miracles until later reflection. They proved to me that God can work miracles through people and things that we come into contact with. Some miracles are bold. Other miracles are seen in tiny gestures from total strangers that leave lasting impressions. I would like to share a couple of these miracles with you.

I survived the terror inflicted on me by Charles and came through it relatively unscathed. Only my ego and my bank account were annihilated. It's worth mentioning that I developed PTSD after our brief marriage. I am lucky and understand that it could have been much worse. I have learned not to trust people for what they tell me. These days

I don't know how many times God helped me through something, and I'm grateful for that.

I trust my intuition. If I feel uneasy about someone I do not pursue a friendship with them. Like the dragonfly, I had to learn to trust myself to make the next step to make the most of this one life here. This is the blessing from the lesson.

Another miracle was just surviving my cardiac arrest. Less than 10% who have a cardiac arrest are revived. My EMTs were volunteers in a small rural town of around 900 people. I was the town of Arena's "First Life Saved" with their newly acquired defibrillator. God also blessed us with fantastic neighbors who brought food for my family while I recovered. Many of whom I'd never met before. I realized how fortunate I was to be alive!

More recently, my son asked me to drive him to Iowa to look at a motorcycle. I somehow knew it would be a memorable experience, though I didn't know why. We drove to Iowa, where Brody inspected the bike, decided to buy it, and I followed him home to be sure nothing went wrong. Still, I had a deep sense of dread. He wore my husband's motorcycle jacket and, thankfully, a helmet. Everything seemed fine until we neared a stoplight. As it turned yellow, I "felt" Brody hesitate – unsure whether to continue or wait for me. In an instant, the bike and Brody slid into the intersection. Aware of a semitruck quickly approaching behind me, I hit my hazard lights and begged God not to let the truck run over my son. Miraculously, the driver saw my lights and instinctively moved into the next lane. Brody was badly shaken, but I knew I had just witnessed another miracle – he was alive and unharmed, except for his pride.

My body underwent a true transformation. I had struggled with many health issues that I believe came about as a result of trauma throughout my life. One health issue I struggled with was a mass in my liver. Doctors monitored it for years by viewing CT scans every six months. Three years ago I received an email from my Hepatologist stating that she was discharging me from hepatology. They could no longer see a mass anywhere on the past two scans. The mass had simply vanished. I was grateful that I didn't have to continue worrying about my liver. I didn't really understand how special that was until I told my general practitioner doctor about my being discharged. His smile lit up the room. He said things like this rarely happen. I knew it was God in action.

Everything in my life seemed to finally be coming together as it should. My health was improving. I continued working out and eating healthy. One day I was visiting a local fruit stand near my home. I was the only customer at the time. I approached Peggy, the woman who ran the stand, with some grapefruit, garlic, and mandarin oranges I wanted to purchase. We started talking about the weather. She had remembered seeing me during the summer when Bryon and I stopped there while we were out on our motorcycle. I thanked her for the produce and headed out of the store. As I was leaving I heard her coming up behind me. "Excuse me," she said. I turned around and noticed that she had something in her hand. I held my hand out to her and she dropped a tiny little metal frog into my hand. She said, "I think you should have this." I was very moved by her kind gesture. "Oh a lucky frog, I will treasure it always. Thank you!" I continued out to my car clutching the little frog. I wanted to do something for her so I grabbed a couple of my poetry books and took them inside for her. As I handed her the books she threw her arms around me and gave me a big hug. She was the embodiment of pure love. A gift from God in the flesh. Three days later I was rushed into emergency surgery for a nasty infection that occurred from a surgery four months earlier. I truly believe that Peggy and her lucky frog were my angel. I am still here today!

I have had a spiritual awakening since my surrender to God. I feel Him all around me. I enjoy exploring nature and being with animals. I believe my spirit is in tune with the universe, something I never thought I'd ever achieve. On one occasion last summer I asked God to send me a dragonfly. I'd watched a Youtube video of a woman swimming in a pool; she would hold her hand up and a dragonfly would land on her hand. I thought it was incredible and I wanted to experience the same thing.

Like most things these days, I forgot about my request. Days passed. Then one day I was standing in my pool when Bryon came out to the pool to talk to me about a minor issue. Something caught my attention in the corner of my eye. No way... I asked Bryon if he saw what I was seeing? There, in the palm of my hand, was a tiny teal damselfly. Close enough to an actual dragonfly for me!! I told Bryon that I asked God for a

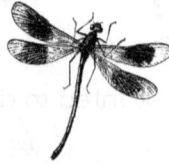

God's Grace

Thank you God for the gift of another day.
I wouldn't change a thing or have it any other way.

I am off to help those who are struggling with living alone.
By doing simple chores or helping them with their phones.

I wonder how my life will be when I reach their age.
I listen intently as they tell their stories; it's my way to engage.

They share memories about their
family members who are now gone.
Learning about all their hardships and
difficulties inspires me to go on.

I am gloriously happy with my life today.
I owe it to God's grace for leading the way.

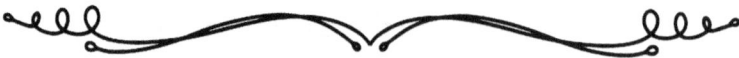

dragonfly and He had answered. Both of us were in awe. Tears of gratitude filled my eyes. I think Bryon was deeply affected also. I thanked God repeatedly. I was satisfied, but He wasn't done with me yet.

My best friend Dianna and I had made plans for her to bring her grandson to my house to swim. I set some time aside in my crazy schedule so we could hang out for a bit in between my clients. I had three hours to swim with them and eat pizza. I hurried through my first client and raced home to meet them. We were set to meet at 11 am. At 11:20 am I texted Dianna to see how much longer she might be. She arrived around noon. Dianna has always been chronically late. I am used to it, but an hour late really pissed me off that day. I didn't want to explode on her in front of her grandson, so I told them to get into their suits and I would be out in a minute. I wanted to compose myself, my rage had been triggered. They headed to the pool and I put a pizza in the oven. Once it was cooked I took it out to the pool for us to eat. The little guy mentioned it was too crispy for him. I asked him to repeat himself as I didn't understand "Whinese." I was being a sarcastic smart-ass. Dianna was not amused, but at that time I really didn't care. I was made to feel like my time meant nothing.

A few days passed and Dianna called me. I was driving to my client's house and parked in front of his apartment. She had been reflecting on our pool date and needed to clear the air. I have never heard her so mad. She reamed my butt. I guess

I deserved it, but then I went on to explain why my behavior was so out of the ordinary. That her tardiness had triggered the feeling of unworthiness in me and led me to become enraged. I told her that I was actually very restrained during their visit.

While I was talking to her I heard something hit my windshield. When I looked up I saw a large golden dragonfly hovering in front of me. I blurted out to Dianna that this gorgeous dragonfly was hitting the windshield right in front me. I believed it was another sign from God. He didn't want us fighting. I fumbled with my phone, trying to get a picture so she could see it. I didn't know you can't take a picture with a phone while talking on it. It flew away just as quickly as it appeared. As I was reminding her of the significance of the dragonfly it reappeared and returned – with a friend. I sat in my car as the two dragonflies danced before my windshield with tears streaming down my face as she and I cried together.

We promised ourselves that day to never fight again. God worked his magic and our 50 year friendship not only survived, but I believe it helped us to thrive! I value our friendship deeply. Dianna has been one of my friends who has been with me through all the difficult times in my life. She has always allowed me to be authentically me. I never had to put on a facade or be anything that I am not. Dianna is the epitome of friendship. I am blessed to know her.

My job sent me to Andrea to help her with some household chores. Andrea is a cancer survivor/patient. The doctors had given her months to live yet she is still here many years later. She has a very calming presence about her. She is very knowledgeable about the Bible. I don't recall how we came about it, but she offered to teach me the Bible when I visited her. I quickly accepted her offer and I have been learning loads from her. She was exactly what I needed so I wasn't intimidated by it. I look forward to our weekly visits together. I think of her as my friend and not just another client. God is bringing me the right people. Seek and Ye shall find as they say!

God truly loves all of us. He wants the best for each of us. Anything is possible if you believe. Have you experienced miracles of your own? Lean on your faith when you are struggling and God will help you as well. Six years ago I would never have believed the changes in my life today. I wouldn't have thought that I would be able to work and share my stories with others. God made it all possible. He can help you too if you just ask him into your heart. I encourage you to give it a try. Knowing God now certainly makes me a believer!

When you pay attention and are open for growth, you can learn lessons from even the worst tragedy.

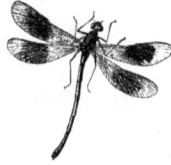

Resilience

What does resilience mean to me?
The ability to rise from struggles with dignity.

I have been knocked down and yet I stand tall.
Being resilient is my superpower after all.

I have survived everything up until today.
I have so much to learn, and I'm doing it my own way.

There were days I wondered if I would make it through.
I practiced gratitude when I didn't know what else to do.

I surrendered my struggles to my higher power.
He gifted me with resilience to help me pass the hours.

It's the strength I gained in facing my fears.
Resilience is rising again in spite of the tears.

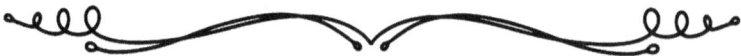

Resilience to Self Love

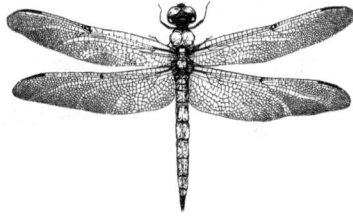

During my recovery from alcohol these past six years I have developed a love of words. I love learning the origins and meanings of words. Resilience is one of the words I was drawn to recently. I recently Googled it to find out the definition: the capacity to withstand or to recover quickly from difficulties; toughness. Another definition: the ability of a substance or object to spring back into shape; elasticity.

I imagined a wad of Silly Putty being stretched out over and over again. Even after being mangled, twisted, and mushed, repeatedly, it still remains Silly Putty. No matter what you do to Silly Putty it always bounces back. I related to its resilience. My faith helped me to become resilient.

Resilience isn't taught to us as children (except for maybe the dysfunctionally resilient things we were told, like "quit your crying or I'll give you something to cry about" or "just take it"). We don't really study resilience; it is more something we become by enduring tough things in life. I had never really given resilience much thought before, but I knew I admired those who had it. While I was reflecting on my life for this book, I was able to see that I had indeed been gifted resilience. I am fascinated how the gift of resilience evolved for me. Resilience is a painful process to endure, yet coming through it brings growth and understanding.

As a child I was sent to Grandma's farm every summer for three months. As much as I loved being there, I missed my parents. Yet when we returned back home to them, I couldn't wait to go back to the farm. I guess that started me down the path of wanting what I couldn't have.

Grandma always made me apologize for anything. Even if Mom started it. Standing up to Mom was always wrong, even when Mom was drunk and stupid. I had to apologize even when I didn't do anything wrong. I took behaviors from people I didn't deserve. So, I became a people pleaser. This led to me constantly being let down by people I trusted with no option but to fail or rise up again. The spirit of resilience was burning inside me. It was ignited when I wanted justice for things that were done to me. It backfired because I wanted "justice" that never came. Now I "step into it" rather than playing small. I didn't want to be perceived as being "tough" – my sister owned that.

I compared my family life to those of my friends, always yearning for that perfect family I saw on TV. I believed that someday my parents would love me. I quickly learned that absence makes the heart grow fonder. We mastered the long distance love affair. It was great while we were apart but upon returning we awoke to the reality of life. My parents were incapable of ever being supportive or involved in our lives. I am grateful that my grandmother took the lead in my life. She was instrumental in teaching me to forgive. I forgive them today because I believe they did the best they could. This journey has taught me that I knew very little about what made them the way that they were. I do not know their whole stories, only the few things they shared with me.

My resilience is the result of grit and grace throughout my life. I was never one to just accept things at face value. I had to do things my way. Right or wrong, my parents lack of care urged me to stand up and protect myself and Tracy the best that I could. We were tragically left to our own devices. Each year we were handed over to airport staff to head up to the farm. We were left unattended for several hours on layovers. Today that would be unthinkable with the child trafficking going on today.

When I was 14 and bought the airline ticket with my birthday money to go to the farm, I had to endure the consequences of my actions at a very young age. My family never came to get me or sent for me. They didn't seem to care.

This taught me that no one was coming to save me. I had to take responsibility for my life, my health, and my beliefs about myself.

I'd never been taught the importance of setting goals. I searched for love to fill the void in my life. Unfortunately that included getting involved in relationships that cost me dearly. Surviving childhood molestation, domestic violence, rape, and financial ruin – yet I remained strong. Coming back from a cardiac arrest, subsequent heart attack, liver mass, and lung nodules, I realized I had survived everything life had thrown at me. I epitomized resilience! God's grace got me through the tough times.

There were days I struggled to get out of bed. I prayed to die. I wondered where all my friends went. With my family gone I wondered if I would ever find happiness. I began a quest to love myself. I needed to heal. I wanted peace. I was tired of running from life, running from myself.

Desperate to understand myself, I dove more into why I was here. I learned recently that we are all one energy. Our actions have reactions. It stems from vibration and frequencies. When I am in alignment, my life flows nicely – I am happy, energetic, and in a positive mood. When I am out of alignment, things get chaotic – I become emotional and edgy. I can visualize the flow of how I would like my life to be. I have learned that if I try too hard to achieve something that doesn't resonate with my energy it never works. Even if I fail I will continue to try to figure out the best way to move forward. That's where being resilient benefits me. Eventually things work out as they should. Resistance and overthinking only complicate things.

When I was at my absolute lowest I contemplated my death. I wanted to die. I locked myself away in my room. I basically laid in bed for over two years. Bryon used to call it the cave. I lived in my bedroom/the cave watching *Law and Order* reruns until I could recite each episode verbatim. My day revolved around watching the same TV shows over and over. I knew what time it was by what TV show was on. I was sick in body, mind, and spirit. Doctors appointments filled my calendar. I had a specialist for everything. I was tired of all of it. I prayed to God to take me home.

I hated myself and my boring predictable life. Drinking alcohol had been my coping method my entire life, but it wasn't relieving my pain or restlessness. It really made everything worse. I didn't enjoy anything. The only time I left the house other than doctor's appointments was to run for cigarettes or alcohol. I drank from morning 'til night. Sleeping was impossible. I stared at the walls. I would visualize what it would look like when I ended my life. I knew that I couldn't take my own life because I knew the destruction it would leave behind for my family. As an empath, whenever I thought about going through with it, the pain I felt for my husband and children always made me change my mind. For those who are struggling, I urge you to play it out all the way through before proceeding. Life is better with you in it than without. God designed each of us with a purpose. When I discovered my purpose, I discovered happiness. God is waiting for you to ask Him into your heart and then He will reveal your purpose to you.

Resilience comes from overcoming difficulties. Instead of becoming a victim of life we must take ownership of the things and make up our minds to overcome whatever it is that is holding you back. I find the serenity prayer helpful.

God, grant me the serenity To accept the things I cannot change, The courage to change the things I can, And the wisdom to know the difference.

That prayer has gotten me through many difficult things in my life. It is commonly used at AA meetings as well. My grandma made a needlepoint of it for me that I reverently hang in my home today.

There comes a time in our life when we have to take responsibility for ourselves. To grow up and own our shortcomings and mistakes. First we acknowledge our baggage and next we take the steps necessary to fix ourselves. For me that meant taking the tiniest of steps each and every day to hold myself accountable. At night when I do an inventory of the day I ask God to forgive me of any sins that

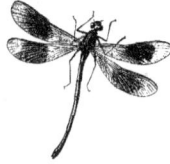

Silly Girl Thing

I guess I am just a silly girl full of dreams.
I am never satisfied or that's how it seems.

I love to be swept off of my feet.
To celebrate life; deflecting defeat.

Romance me, the more elaborate the better.
Use your imagination to celebrate our life together.

I know it's just a silly girl thing,
I love romance and all that it brings.

Whether it's a walk by the river or a picnic in the park.
It just might bring about good times after dark.

Silly girl things always make me smile.
Give it a try, you might just find it's worthwhile.

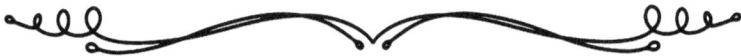

I may have committed during my day, I readily accept that I am an imperfect creature. I give myself to God in obedience and gratitude for what he brings to me. Every day is a new opportunity to be of service to others.

I am able now to extend grace to myself and others. Though I regret harboring the pain I incurred for so long, forgiveness truly released whatever trauma I held onto so desperately for most of my life. I am a different person altogether. I am whole. I am love. I am.

I no longer seek validation from others. I have learned to give myself grace in my quest to understand and love myself. I have befriended the wounded child I tried to drown with rum and Diet Cokes for so many years. Loving myself did not come easily, but it was worth every bit of the work to have the peace I have today. My prayer for those reading is to look deep inside yourself for true understanding of your beliefs. I am grateful for having the resilience to still be here today. The glory goes to our creator, I am just His messenger.

The message is don't ever give up. The voice inside of you telling you that you aren't enough is a lie. It is Satan trying to destroy you. The voice that told me I was unlovable was a liar. That was the devil. Anytime you feel inadequate, unworthy, dispensable, challenge it. Ask yourself: Is it real? Is it kind? Would you talk that way to your friend? If not, it's Satan. Invite God into your life.

My sister Tracy and I both lashed out by hurting ourselves. We couldn't get our parents to love us, why should we love ourselves? We ended up putting ourselves in situations we shouldn't have been in. It was a challenge to get over how worthless I felt, no wonder I made the choices I made.

I started getting sick after my kids were born. The cardiac arrest left me scared and feeling like I was going to die at any moment, which drove me further into my alcohol addiction. I lost my intuition, and trust in myself. I became the illness, the sickness, the disabled person. I became ready to die. Why even try?

> *I surrendered myself to God and He gifted me the strength to continue living when I wanted to die so desperately.*

I'd like to take a moment to remind you that we are here for one another. At my sickest, I alienated myself because I didn't want to burden others. I desperately needed my friends, and when they disappeared it was a wake up call, because I DO need community in my life. It was families (and neighbors) in my earlier life who took us in from time to time. Being alone is bad for your spiritual, mental, and physical health. It is sometimes necessary to go through things alone to get in touch with your spiritual self, to truly understand your soul. And maybe, like it did for me, in that solitude, come into alignment with the Universe, and with God. But consider if your best friend was going to kill themselves, what would you say to them? I wish I'd had a friend to give me a book or whatever it took to get me out of bed. I learned the path to healing is about taking responsibility for making such choices. I also now understand that my mental illness was the result of trauma rather than being a flawed individual. Further, I learned that my physical illnesses have manifested due to trauma I've endured. This is hard work, but it is so worth it!

Addiction

No one sets out to become an addict. I was born into addiction and eventually I became like those I surrounded myself with. Growing up I learned that people liked to drink. They drank when they were happy. They drank when they were sad. They drank when they were mad. They drank when they were anxious. They drank to celebrate. I drank for all those reasons, too, and also to be numb. I wanted to escape from my life. I wanted the pain to end. I wanted to be loved. Eventually I learned that alcohol is a liar. It solved nothing. Alcohol betrayed me as it had betrayed my whole family for generations. Alcohol is a killer. It is poison. It killed my aunt and my sister. It keeps us distracted from life. It tricks us to believe that it brings fun into our boring, predictable lives. It wreaks havoc on families and it destroys dreams. Generations of families fall prey to alcohol. It's cunning and baffling. It wants us to need it. It convinces many of us that we are weak and useless without it.

As a child I swore that I would never be like my parents. Growing up I remember nagging them to quit smoking. Such a filthy, stinky habit. I hated the way they smelled. Did it stop me from using cigarettes as a teenager? Nope. I got so nauseous from smoking I lost 25 pounds when I started. I used it to lose weight and got addicted. The stupidest thing I ever did was smoke cigarettes. Such a colossal waste of money. Thankfully, after 36 years I quit that habit over five years ago!

Alcohol and cigarettes were a choice I made. Let's talk about prescription meds. In my late teens I was prescribed antidepressants for the first time. Elavil, then Prozac. The doctors were readily supplying me with sleep and anxiety meds. I began to depend on these for major mood swings and sleepless nights. Living in Vegas, crowds would bother me. I worked in jobs requiring me to frequent the casinos. As an empath I now understand that my body was having a heightened response to all the chaos and energy of the crowds. I thought the feelings and energy that I experienced at the time were mine. I came to accept that I was very moody. I chalked it up to PMS and I thought the pills would be helpful at managing all the crazy feelings I was dealing with. I started using them for everything. Stressful day at work, pop a benzo.

Slam a pot of coffee or caffeine pills and now I was ready to party and drink most of the night, then come home and take a sleeping pill or down a bottle of NyQuil. Are we having fun yet? This was my life for years. The drugs changed but the self destruction did not. As I got older the drugs got better. Marijuana was the least of it. In my twenties I discovered cocaine. Bonanza! It gave me energy, self confidence, and man was I able to get things done. Vegas in the 80s was insane. The nightclubs in Vegas were fantastic. The ambiance, the energy, the music, lights, and so much cocaine. I felt like a supermodel. I became addicted to the atmosphere.

I became addicted to everything: food, men, coke, alcohol, I was never satisfied. It all left me with this emptiness inside. There had to be more to life than this. I yearned for someone to love me. I wanted to be able to just be me. Not some coked up disco queen. I did not have a role model. I needed someone to help me learn to love myself. I could not find love in alcohol, drugs, or men who just wanted to use me. I felt like I deserved better, but I had nowhere to turn. I settled for people who did not deserve me.

It wasn't until I had finally tried everything else that I surrendered to God. I had tried many approaches at living a sober life. A few rehabs, years of therapy, nothing stuck until I was physically, mentally, emotionally, and spiritually bankrupt. My depression after losing my mom, dad, grandma, and sister was horrible. I lived in my bedroom cave with the blinds drawn.

I couldn't stand myself. I was angry at God for sparing my life repeatedly when I wanted to die. I'd had enough of this world. The problem was the immense loss/pain I knew my husband and children would endure if I committed suicide. I loved them more than I hated myself. I had to give my life to God. I recognized the fact that I wasn't able to continue living this way any longer. My faith was strong. I knew if anyone could help me it was God.

On August 29, 2019, I asked my son Brody to drive me to the hospital. I promised him that this would be the last time. I had to check in to the hospital to detox because of my heart condition. They'd have to monitor me as I came off the alcohol. I was sober when I went in. The hospital was not amused when I arrived and announced that I was there to detox. I didn't care. I had nowhere else to go and I had nothing to lose at that point. I was ready this time.

Unfortunately most addicts don't voluntarily decide to get sober. Most of those who I've met in rehab were there because it was court ordered. For whatever reason I denied my drinking problem for the longest time. I never got into trouble with the law, I never got a DUI, or had marital problems. That was for other people. I was sick. I had a heart, lung, liver condition, blah, blah, blah. If people only knew what I had been through then they would understand. No, I was a closet drinker. A stay-at-home mother. I appeared to be fine on the outside. No one knew or attempted to intervene, so I didn't see the harm. I told myself all kinds of things to rationalize my lifestyle. I was a functional alcoholic and in true Dani form, I took it to the extreme. I was lying to myself and I hate liars. I had become just like my mother. I became the best self loathing person on the planet.

Finally God said "Enough!!" for me. I now know that it was God who gave me the strength and resilience to change. My stubbornness and beliefs about myself began to change. I realized that my heart had hardened over the years. I had become cynical and bitter about life. God helped to soften me. He proved to me that I am worthy of love. He taught me how to heal myself in all ways. I started to take care of myself again. Journaling was instrumental in my understanding myself. I practiced forgiveness of others who had hurt me. People I'd never get apologies from. I let go of the anger and was now dealing with years of buried rage. I learned to give myself grace. I now identify myself as a beautiful disaster. I accept my flaws and imperfections. I do things "messy" and that's okay. I accept that I don't have to fix everything for everyone. I go with the flow instead of resisting change. I learned that failure is success in practice.

Addicts have one thing in common – they have unresolved trauma that must be dealt with. Our healthcare system wants to throw pills at us to deal with it. The pills don't work. They all have unwanted and life changing side effects from tardive dyskinesia, to massive weight gain, to loss of sex drive, to mood shifts. Addicts also encounter judgment when seeking treatment. Until something major changes, this is how it will be. No one makes the choice to become an addict. We must bring empathy back into our emergency rooms. No one deserves to be looked down upon for struggling.

Life today is better than I ever dreamed was possible for me. Don't give up!! Honor yourself for making it this far. Please know it is never too late. I was almost 50 when I decided to change, so age is no reason. I am grateful to be six years off booze and five and a half off cigarettes!

Look inward and reevaluate those beliefs you have about yourself. Are they relevant? Are they true? Would you talk to your best friend the way you talk to yourself? If you are unsure, ask God into your life. When you establish a relationship with God your life is guaranteed to change. I am living my best life and I can finally be authentically me! And you know what? I am not the bad person I believed I was for most of my life. When I am in alignment with the universe it feels amazing. The best part is now I am able to help others who are struggling with the same issues. It is possible for you, too. Believe!

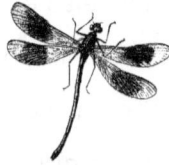

For Today

Keep going when things get rough
Keep going, it'll make you tough.

Look for the lessons when things aren't going your way.
Practice gratitude to get you through the day.

Find your purpose, it will help you feel great.
Do things today; you can no longer wait.

Don't let perfection hold you back.
Be authentically you, even when you feel attacked.

Above all give yourself grace.
Remember to enjoy the journey; you're not in a race.

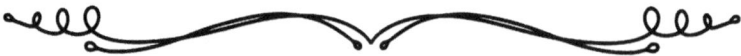

Happiness IS Your Choice

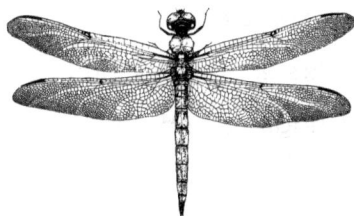

$\mathcal{I}$ often felt like happiness has eluded me throughout my life, and I stayed living under a black cloud for most of it. Bouts of depression wore me out. I thought that was just my luck. I am here to tell you that happiness is a choice. I was so sick of being sick. It was my life. Always running to doctors appointments, never getting better. When I learned about the Law of Attraction I started to practice gratitude. What happened next left me speechless.

When I focused on the positive things in my life, the universe rewarded me by giving me more to be thankful for. Likewise, if I was having a bad day and complained about how terrible everything in my life was, the universe would give me more to bitch about. I focused all my energy on getting healthy. I visualized myself in my perfect body. I visualized myself dancing with a huge smile on my face. I listened to songs that brought me joy. I choose not to watch the news anymore. The negativity would spill over into my day. Instead I choose to listen to daily devotionals and podcasts focusing on becoming the best person I could be. I also did things to improve my mental health. Exercise, meditation, and breathwork help me to calm myself and release negativity. Being an empath, I often take on other people's energy and problems. I can feel if they are in trouble or struggling with something. It is my nature to try to help them. Too often, though, I end up feeling drained and alone once their problems have been resolved. I learned to walk away from people who didn't align with me anymore. I surround myself with like minded people who are interested in bettering themselves and being of service to others.

I remember to pray each night and thank God for the gift of each new day. As I pray, I remind myself of how far I have come in the past few years. I am a completely different person than I was before. I dedicate myself to serving others as long as possible. I hope to help people who are struggling with mental health or addiction. We must find a way to normalize having a bad day or a difficult season. By sharing our stories it helps those who are on the fence make the tough decision to get the help they need. Something may resonate with them and inspire them to give it a try.

What I can say about this ordeal is that we must stop blaming others for our shortcomings. We have each experienced things that have caused pain at one time or another. Everyone we encounter has a story. We must stop living as a victim. Take back the control of your life. After my cardiac arrest many of my friends stayed away from me. I retreated into my room and deeper into my mind, overthinking everything.

My illness was foremost on my mind at all times. I became a victim of heart disease. I lived in fear of my next cardiac event. I alienated myself because I believed no one could possibly understand what I was going through. I did not want anyone's pity. Alone, at my own doing, I stayed in bed only getting out to make dinner for the family. I struggled with immense depression that I now understand is common following a cardiac arrest. I was on every medication offered. At one time I was taking over 30+ pills daily. I stayed sick. Each new pill I prayed would bring relief from my pain and depression. I prayed for help that never came. Then I made a change – I prayed for strength. God answered my prayers with other challenges that made me stronger. I prayed for courage to endure and I gained resilience. I prayed for answers and I gained wisdom and understanding. I prayed for my depression to be lifted and God revealed my purpose. I started to gain understanding of my relationship with God. I know He has special plans for each of us. For the first time in my life I finally felt worthy and loved. I understood why I had been able to come through every challenge in my life. It was through God's grace. He was responsible for it all.

Everything that surrounds us was created in His unique design. Everything has a specific purpose, including people. We are meant to function as a community. Each is able to be of service within the community, in their own unique way. Together we are stronger. I have come to understand that during our lifetime forces have driven us further away from our Lord and Savior, Jesus Christ. We need to unite as people and stop the needless divide. We must get back to our roots and remember our why. Everything in our lives is possible only because of God. We are to represent Him as good Christians who follow the Golden Rule. *Do unto others as you shall have done unto you.* That's it. Simple. Yet so many of us are so caught up in our lives that we often forget how all of it is possible. We are too rushed and forget to live in the present. We quickly put off our dreams for "someday." Unfortunately, those somedays never come and we become bitter. We are filled with regrets of letting time slip through our hands waiting for somedays. Understanding my relationship with God has taught me that He wants us all to be happy. He loves all of us. We are responsible for not recognizing God's gift of life. We are already living in Heaven, folks. There is nothing that God did not think of. His designs are perfect.

Have you ever truly looked at a dragonfly? The wings are like stained glass, shimmering and paper thin. You wouldn't think those beautifully intricate wings could allow them to hover and fly at great speed. Those beautiful creatures evolved from a grubby little larva surviving in the muck of a pond. But they had to go through a wondrous process of metamorphosis to grow to become the adult dragonfly. I can relate to this transformation. I have been through a lot in life. My faith led me back to God. From there I have been given an understanding of God's perfect plan. I had to put my faith in His hands and then allow myself to follow His guidance.

God waits for us to invite him into our lives. He does not force himself into our lives, he must be invited. Once you understand His true love for each of us, you are instantly hooked. His love is unlike any other. Pick up a Bible and look for understanding. It's time to heal and grow. Don't waste another day. You are worthy of happiness. Only you know what would bring you joy. I say go for it. Our days are fleeting. Enough time has been wasted with sadness. Give your worries to God and claim your happiness today!

I have learned a lot recently about happiness. I used to believe that happiness was the opposite of depression. I discovered the cure for depression is purpose. Once you figure out your purpose, happiness will follow. It requires a lot of self evaluation and reflection. And soul searching to better understand yourself. What are your dreams? What would make you happy? So many people have forgotten their dreams. You need to visualize yourself being happy. What would you do if you could? Once you figure out what would bring you happiness, envision yourself already doing whatever it is you think would bring you joy. Then act as if happiness is already yours. Happiness will follow. Unfortunately our dreams have been replaced with responsibilities for families, jobs, or other things. We become stuck in an unfulfilling cycle. Work, sleep, and repeat. Life becomes dull when you can predict each day.

We need to look at our beliefs from time to time to see if the things we keep telling ourselves are actually relevant. Often you will see your beliefs stem from your culture, society, or religion. We have a tendency to value the opinions of others more than we value our own. One reason for that is familiarity. Another is fear. It's more comfortable to just believe what you've always believed than to actually challenge yourself to see it is still relevant today. I encourage everyone to check their beliefs from time to time. Then step out of your comfort zone and learn something new. Take up a new hobby, or learn a new language; just do something out of the ordinary and see how it makes you feel.

People don't like discomfort, so they never change and they remain stuck and unhappy. It's easier to believe that happiness just eluded you. We need to get comfortable with being uncomfortable. We have become a weaker society through our evolution. We must get curious about why we believe the things we do.

We have become a generation of people who want everything now. In our rush for fame, wealth, or status, etc., we must be mindful that the struggles we endure help bring forward the best versions of ourselves. Growth is a process that takes time and many don't see any need to change until it's too late.

I am here to tell you happiness is a choice. Yep, that's right, I said it. I believe it. As a person who struggled with depression throughout my life, I thought I was unhappy because of my health or circumstances. My mentality was "you'd be miserable, too, if you had my health problems…" I became a victim. A victim of my life, of myself, a victim of everything. Poor me. I wallowed in self pity. It was not good. I somehow believed that happiness was out of reach for me.

How to Achieve Happiness

Look for the lesson when a day is difficult
(keep it simple at first)

Own your bullshit
(acknowledge your actions)

Stop living in denial
(blaming others for current life)

Don't fall into victimhood
(even health is in your hands to fix)

I have since realized it was in my control all along. My mindset always saw the negative in things. I challenged myself to find the good when I started to practice gratitude. Gratitude was eye opening. I realized that I have everything I need already. God had provided me with a beautiful life in the country. I have the world's greatest husband who has tolerated everything I have put him through. He loves me for me. He blessed me with the family I always wanted. Are things perfect? Hell no! But that's ok, because neither am I. I look for glimmers in my daily life; reminders from the universe that God thought of everything. I am fine just as I am because I was created by God's design.

I look for the good every day. I am aware of the negativity in our world. I try to avoid the news and people who want to bring me down. I don't dwell on anything that is out of my control. If something is affecting my energy negatively I give it to God. He gives me strength. He gives me free will to choose whether I have a good day or a bad day. I will always choose to have a good day. There is so much beauty to be found in people and experiences, why not look for the good? Then choose to find something to make yourself happy.

Acknowledge what is not serving you and then take the steps to make the changes you need to make to find your happiness. First and foremost, you must embrace change. Then you change your mindset. Move from complaining, and being stuck, and look for positive things and build on that so we can make change with purpose. You must condition yourself to look for the positive, and happiness will follow.

I always believed happiness was never in the cards for me.... I felt I had everything I needed, but actually, I lacked for little, but wasn't happy. Things would not bring happiness, it had to come from within. And only then was I able to experience true happiness.

Psalms 23:6
Surely goodness and loyal love will pursue me all the days of my life,
And I will dwell in the house of the Lord for all of my days.

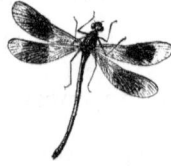

Stay the Course

If you want all your dreams to come true
You must start first by working on you.

Let go of all the baggage from your past.
Be mindful of your time because it goes by so fast.

Envision yourself living the life of your dreams.
Happiness will follow; it's as easy as it seems.

When you begin to take action to finally get things done
Know that challenges that you encounter will be part of the fun.

Slowly you will see your dreams come into fruition.
You will begin to acknowledge your own intuition.

Stay the course and you will see
Everything you imagine will come to be.

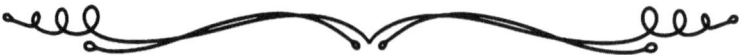

Gratitude to Find Joy

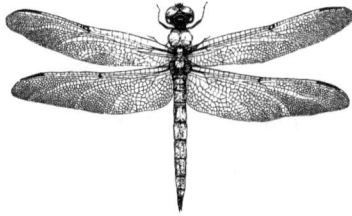

When I began to practice gratitude my life changed instantly. I quickly realized that I've had everything I'd ever wanted right in front of me. I have a husband who adores me, who has stuck by me through all the tough times. He breathed for me when I died during my cardiac arrest. He went to every doctor's appointment with me. He stepped up when I needed time to heal by tending to the children and maintaining his business as well. He never complained. He allowed me time to figure out what I needed to do to become a better mother and person. He believed in me when I couldn't accept or love myself. He's given me a stable home and a beautiful family complete with a bonus son! Bryon has been my biggest supporter and my best friend. God knew what he was doing when he brought us together.

I may not have been a perfect mother. I do believe my children have been the ultimate gift from God. Being their mother has been the best and the hardest thing that I've ever done. I now understand unconditional love. I didn't hide my struggles from them. I wanted them to understand the challenges one can face through the years. I want them to understand that it's not necessary to be perfect. It's through our failures that we learn and grow. I am grateful that they witnessed my faults and my recovery! I encourage them to look within themselves to find their unique purpose in life. I want my children to be happy. I hope to lead them to God. Each of us is responsible for becoming the best versions of ourselves. To do so we must understand why we are the way we are. Then once we've acknowledged our shortcomings can we take steps to improve ourselves. No more blaming others, no more victimhood, only focusing on the goal of self improvement.

I'm grateful for these past 21 bonus years. I've grown so much. I'm grateful for the struggles and the valuable lessons I learned. I couldn't see it at the time, but those struggles were exactly what I needed. I am grateful for every day. I take nothing for granted any more. I relish fun times with friends and family.

I do everything I can to stay healthy. I take breaks when needed. I understand that my body needs rest even when my brain has other ideas. I am more accepting that I've been through a lot in life and that I am a work in progress. I realize that it's up to me to take care of myself. No one is coming to save me. Only God is my redeemer. I am able to extend grace to myself these days. I am a perfectly imperfect sinner, yet I am still loved by God.

Practicing gratitude keeps me mindful of the blessings in my life. Through gratitude practice I realized that it was the little things that brought me much of my joy. Phone calls from old friends. Observing bees pollinating my flowers. Playing Frisbee with my dog. Walking in the woods. I look for things to be grateful for each day. Since adopting this belief my attitude improved and became positive. The negativity fell by the wayside.

These days I thank God each morning for opening my eyes. I appreciate the gift of another day to experience and seek out the little glimmers that surround me. A beautiful sunrise, a warm cup of mushroom coffee, and puppy kisses. I thank God for it all. On the less-than-ideal days, I look for the lessons and thank God for those as well. I value my relationship with Him these days. He fills my soul with love and for that I am forever grateful. I no longer live with fear for the future – and that brings me confidence that I didn't have before. I live with faith knowing that God is with me always. Faith in God reminds me of His love for us. I know He will continue to use me to help others, for I was designed for this. By discovering my purpose, the joy I had always been longing for has finally been found.

Exercises to Develop Gratitude

Gratitude Journal. Write down three things you're grateful for each day. Be specific and try to find new things regularly. I find it helpful to use stickers with inspirational sayings; they brighten the journal and opened up different ideas for me to write about in my journal.

"Best Part of the Day" Reflection. At the end of the day, recall the best moment and appreciate why it mattered. Before I go to sleep I like to remember the positive things that occurred during the day. I fall asleep with a smile of gratitude.

Gratitude Letter. Write a heartfelt letter to someone who has positively impacted your life (even if you don't send it). Gratitude letters are a great way to thank someone and help us to be kind. Who doesn't like to be thanked?

Gratitude Walk. Take a walk and intentionally notice and appreciate nature, people, or small joys around you. Incorporate this into your daily routine. Stop and notice your surroundings. Look at the clouds, smell the flowers, listen to the birds singing. Live in the present moment.

Meditation on Gratitude. Sit quietly and focus on things you're grateful for, visualizing them vividly. Mediation is a challenge for this overthinking brain of mine. Patience with oneself is helpful. Practice makes perfect.

Gratitude Jar. Write things you're grateful for on slips of paper and collect them in a jar to read later. Put prayers or verses into a Bible jar with different colored strips related to different emotions. This is also a great way to learn Bible scripture.

Express Thanks Daily. Make it a habit to thank someone sincerely each day. I can't underscore enough how this has to be a DAILY practice. It is very rewarding to bring joy into someone's life when they are alone and desolate.

Share Gratitude at Meals. If you eat with others, take turns sharing one thing you're grateful for before eating. We must thank God for providing us with life sustaining meals.

Gratitude Buddy. Partner with someone to regularly share things you're grateful for via text or conversation. A fun way to share the good things in your life. Be aware that not everyone will share in your happiness. Share with those who are truly happy for your successes.

Reframe Challenges. When facing difficulties, find one lesson or silver lining in the situation. Always look for the lesson. How can I do this better?

Appreciation Lists. Pick a specific category (e.g., "People who helped me grow" or "Small comforts I enjoy") and list things within it. Helpful for when you are feeling low. You will see you don't have it as bad as you envision. Look to find the good, never to compare to someone else. Comparison will rob you of joy.

Gratitude Visualization. Imagine what life would be like without certain comforts, then appreciate them more deeply. Did you sleep in a bed last night? Did you have clean water? Have you ever imagined what it would be like to be homeless? We are blessed in so many ways.

Nightly Prayer. This can be of thanks for protection, and for the events that occurred that day. Prayer of thanks for the glimmers throughout the day.

Believe in yourself. What is it that you want to achieve or do with your life? Challenge yourself to step out of your comfort zone. Take some chances in life. Try an open mic night, or painting class, whatever you think might bring you joy. Just do it. Fear of failure often holds us back. Once we complete these challenges we realize they weren't so scary after all.

Set goals for yourself. Take tiny steps to move forward each day. Practice gratitude for your progress.

Gratitude affirmations. Today I am grateful for being strong, everything is always working out for me. Today I am thankful for the food that makes me healthy. I am thankful for the people that God brings into my life. I am strong and healthy because of God's grace.

Reading the Bible. I can't tell you how many times I have picked up a Bible only to get discouraged trying to comprehend what I had just read. The difficult names of cities and towns always overwhelmed me just trying to pronounce them correctly. I got so hung up on the tiny details. I felt guided to retry again once I found a friend who understood it. Her understanding and patience helped me to see the overlap between the days back then and our current times. I am fascinated by that relevance that had eluded me until now. You can't help but feel gratitude for Jesus and His ultimate sacrifice for all of us.

Practice Breathwork. Learning to slow down your breath can be so helpful to your mind. We hold a lot in with our breathing... when we learn to control it, it relaxes our nervous system. I take in a deep breath, hold it for the count of four and then fully exhale and this helps me to calm down when I feel overwhelmed.

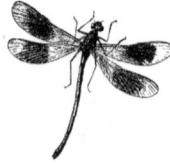

Lead with Love

May I share my story with you?
I feel it may help in whatever you do.

Like many others I have survived a lot of trauma.
These days I do my best to avoid any drama.

I must testify to everyone about my savior.
He saved my life and forgave my past behaviors.

My physical pain and mental health won't hold me back.
I refuse to surrender, even when I am under an attack.

I urge you to give your heart and soul to God above.
Forgive those who have hurt you;
remember to always Lead with Love.

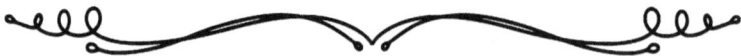

Faith

My faith has sustained me through my difficulties. I've always been an overthinker. I was always curious about things, people, nature, and generally in search of meaning. I love to witness the interactions between things. Faith kept me believing that surely a God who could create a world with such forethought must have a reason for me, too. I was never a person who set goals. Heck, I couldn't even achieve any New Year's resolutions. I was never taught the importance of having a dream and then pursuing it. I always did whatever I pleased. Sometimes to my detriment. Life has shown me repeatedly that God's plan is always best.

It wasn't until I surrendered my life completely to God that He revealed His plan for me. I started following my intuition. My faith made it possible. I started being led to people who inspired me to improve myself. I took ownership of my health. I have trusted doctors to heal me, but it never worked out well. I could no longer continue to take pills with all kinds of nasty side effects. I started researching supplements for my various conditions. I contacted a naturopath who helped me know which ones would give me the best results. I started to move my body. Exercise helped me to stay out of my head and to burn calories to lose weight. Consistency was key. I had a friend work out with me to hold me accountable. Discipline was imperative, and showed results quickly. When I was injured or sick, my faith inspired me to rest briefly and not use it as an

The way to gratitude is to have faith and then you'll start to recognize the miracles.

excuse to give up. Faith showed me that God was making a way for me. I found when I followed God's protocol, life was great. My faith in God has made it possible. His love for me pulled me out of the darkness that I struggled with for most of my life. Saying the Child's Prayer nightly reminded me that God had always been there for me. I've been saying it since I was a child. Grandma made me memorize it and gifted me a plaque with it written on it. She made me memorize it. It was the best gift ever for it instilled my faith in God. I am eternally grateful to her for that gift. Now I understand He was making it possible for me to help others.

God opened my eyes to the imbalance of the world – including challenges that raising an Autistic son presents. It was as if He removed the blinders that had kept me unaware of the pure evil that is happening in our world. I could see things in a new light. As an empath I like to fix things – people, situations, world problems, etc. When I had this awakening I wanted to be the one to fix everything. If you have known me long you know that when I care about something I go all in to remedy things. My mind gets flooded with solutions for change. It causes me to become very overwhelmed at times. Since my surrender to God, I realized that He wasn't showing me the evil in this world for me to fix it, but merely to be aware of how dark the world has become. It is beyond my control but I must be aware. I can be a light for others in their dark times.

Faith gives me the ability to believe in things that I cannot see. I believe that God is always working things for my favor because he wants all of us to be happy. Faith helped me see the happiness in front of me. Faith restored the hope I had lost. It gave hope to the hopeless, as they say. My faith tells me now that I have nothing to fear. God is much stronger than anything that comes my way. As a person once overwhelmed with anxiety I now understand that I created the fear of those things in my mind. I take responsibility for that and my faith tells me God's always got my back.

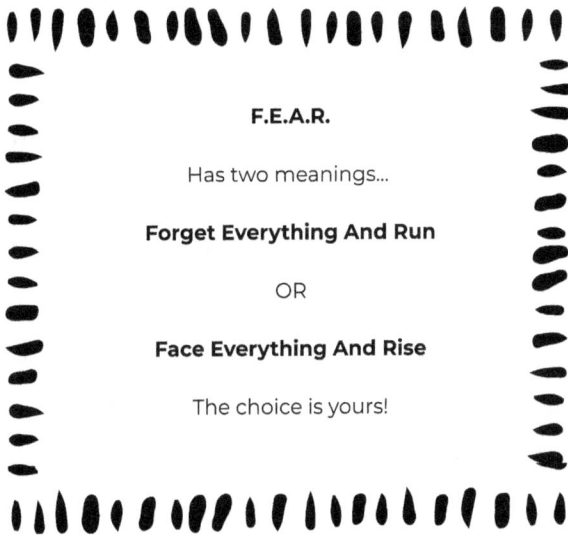

F.E.A.R.

Has two meanings...

Forget Everything And Run

OR

Face Everything And Rise

The choice is yours!

(From Beautiful Disaster Card bdrocks.com)

Our minds can cause us to do all kinds of things that aren't beneficial for us. Satan and the likes use fear as a way to keep us apart from God. I once thought drinking was great fun. I longed to be the life of the party. My constant desire for validation ruled my life and was ultimately responsible for my poor health. I was afraid when I quit drinking that no one would like me and I'd be considered boring. That was all the things my brain was telling me. I drank for much longer than I should have. I made myself sick. I went through pancreatitis twice. The last time they wanted me to have my children come to the hospital to say their goodbyes. My faith told me it wasn't goodbye. It caused me to surrender. It was the intervention that I needed. Being close to death brings us closer to God.

My stubbornness had met its match. God never abandoned me. He was with me through all my difficulties even when I challenged him. My troubles arose because I turned *away* from him. God gifts each of us with free will. I was free to do as I pleased. Remember, however, that each action has a consequence. My party girl days resulted in fatty liver disease, pre-cirrhosis, and a liver mass. I went all in and added cigarette smoking to the list of the ways to kill myself. Ending up with lung issues and shortness of breath at all times. For kicks I ate to comfort my sick and misunderstood self. Blossoming up to a full 300 pounds. While meds added weight, ultimately it was me and my lack of discipline that packed on the weight. My faith in God opened my eyes to my role in my health. He showed me the ways to heal. He gifted me with humility and a desire to improve myself. In time, I addressed the things I needed to fix – one by one. It's been a process of learning to trust my intuition as he guides me toward healing myself.

I am still and probably will always be a work in progress – a beautiful disaster. It fits me to a tee. I have aged and through it I gained wisdom. And with that wisdom I am empowered to support others on their journey towards self love and acceptance.

Hebrews 11:1
Faith is the assured expectation of what is hoped for, the evident demonstration of realities that are not seen.

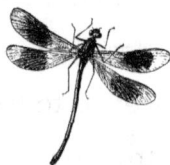

Learning to Love Yourself

Escape the negative self-talk
Get outside and take a walk

Being in nature is healthy for you
Breathe in fresh air; expel anything that is bothering you.

Perhaps being near the water could help to clear your mind?
Go somewhere new, you never know what you may find.

Take some time to just relax
To decompress and put an end to those panic attacks.

Try stepping out of your comfort zone every once in a while.
You might actually discover something
that enriches your smile!

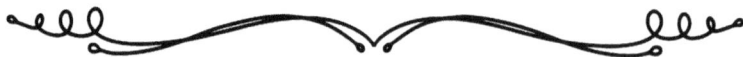

How do I Love Me?

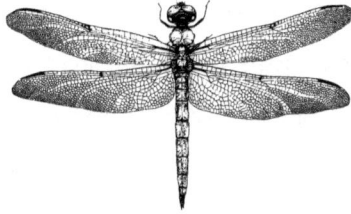

Loving myself did not come easy. My entire life I have had a critical inner dialogue with myself. I was unlovable, a burden, ugly, fat, unstable, over sensitive, etc. I straight up hated myself. I was taught that I only mattered for my looks. My looks got me whatever I needed to survive. My life was a phony facade of how I believed things were supposed to be. Growing up I was taught to be seen and not heard. To always look my best. Presenting myself as capable and worthy in whatever scenario I was in. I always felt like a fraud. Only to retreat to my bed at night wondering the true meaning of life. It all left me feeling empty. I had been involved in too many abusive relationships. I allowed people to disrespect me. I felt I somehow deserved it. I was abused and somehow felt that it was my fault.

I was a child who needed help yet no one came. My parents knew what had happened to me yet did nothing. No one got me any professional help in dealing with feelings after being molested by Don. I took it to mean that I was unimportant, I was branded a filthy minded liar. I believe that was easier than getting me the help I so desperately needed. I was disregarded by those who claimed to love me. Unlovable was the message I told myself over and over again.

When I became sick my friends disappeared. I never understood why. I now realize that my sickness reminded them of their own mortality. After my father-in-law died, my brother-in-law actually told me that he was ready to put me in the ground next. Funny thing was I didn't remember him even calling to check on me, knowing I was so close to death.

I had a sort of epiphany, after my surrender to God, that I was holding space for people who could care less about me at all. As someone who always stood up for the underdog, something lit up inside of me and I did a quick inventory of people I allowed into my life. I became very protective of the wounded child inside of me. I needed to establish boundaries so that I wouldn't get hurt as often. I stood up for myself for a change. I deserved better. I didn't know how to love myself, but I was desperate enough to work on it. I knew nobody was coming to rescue me. I had finally had enough self loathing and pity that I was determined to make whatever changes I had to. The fear that kept me paralyzed now changed into determination and I was determined to find joy.

At the advice of my therapist, I started to journal. She instructed me to find three things I liked about myself each day. At first I was very superficial. I liked my hair, my eyes, and my hands. Several weeks later it evolved into something like nice legs, strong hands, and determination. Wait, what was that? Determination? Where did *that* come from?

I started to explore determination. I was very sick for many years – bedridden by my depression and illnesses for two years. It was through my determination that I made the difficult choice to change my life. Determination, that I attribute to God, that I was able to get out of that negative mindset and take the steps to heal. Slowly, I started to emerge as a new, unrecognizable version of myself. I quit drinking alcohol, started exercising, and stopped smoking cigarettes.

I began to research holistic health remedies to heal my damaged body. I was no longer someone who hated myself. I was now a friend to myself. I went from the wounded child self into the empowered woman I am today. I accepted the scars I had been carrying. They are reminders of all the things I have survived. I finally started to take care of myself like I would have done for any of my friends.

Love yourself first before getting into a relationship.

Today I am healthier in all aspects of my life. I own the fact that I am a plus sized gal! I am full of empathy and love for everyone. I am not perfect and I don't claim to be. Fear of failure kept me paralyzed. These days I "do life messy." I try new things. I step out of my comfort zone regularly. I show vulnerability, and trust that God will always protect me. I am able to be authentically me! No more phony facades. I am perfectly imperfect and that's enough for me.

I now love myself completely, by doing so I am able to live with purpose. God has given me an abundance of love so that I can help others who are struggling too. I want for nothing these days. Since I have gained acceptance of myself I realized how blessed I am. God has gotten me through some very tough times. I am grateful for my life today. I live in awe of God's creations. Each day I take time to notice the small things around me. I am eager to begin each day. I no longer look to others in search of validation. The love I have for God sustains me. He gives my peace and understanding. I do not need riches or fame to sustain me. I yearn for tranquility and peace these days.

On difficult days I look for the lessons. I know God is working on something better for me. I no longer live in fear of being accepted. God has shown me I matter and I am loved. Better yet God taught me how to love myself, to me that is priceless. Now I can love others fully and completely having healed my tattered heart. It feels great to be alive these days.

Learning to love myself was a long process. I had to find a way to value myself. Growing up was challenging because I had repeatedly learned that I didn't matter. I had interpreted that to mean I was unlovable or unworthy. Actually it was unlearning many things I believed about myself. After I became sober all my insecurities came to the surface. Previously, these beliefs were the reasons I sabotaged my sobriety. This time was going to be different because I had discovered my purpose in life. That gave me something to focus on instead of my own insecurities.

I knew that God created me for this very reason and he gave me the strength to see it through.

I started finding speakers and authors who resonated with my ideas and goals. Gregg Braden talked about three important life lessons. The first was that we are divine beings. I agree wholeheartedly with him on this. During my quest to love myself I dove into my spiritual beliefs. I have learned that we truly are capable of creating our own destiny based on our purpose. Once we tap into our spiritual connection with God, our divine self will be revealed. Second, we must love fearlessly. This is what being human is all about. Loving our neighbors and helping people in our communities. Much strife is going on in this world. Do what you can to be of service to others. It's very rewarding. People are lonely, depressed, and defeated. I was too.

God doesn't want that for us. There is much turmoil in this world. He wants us to be aware of it. He wants us to do better. He wants us to follow the teachings of His son Jesus Christ. Do unto others as you shall have done to you. Walk around in someone else's shoes. Think of what they are dealing with. Then lead with love to help them when you can. Other times pray for those who are struggling so that they may find their way to God through Jesus. Above all, if you can't be kind, then say nothing because words can leave permanent scars. And, lastly, remember goodness with gratitude. I can't stress this enough: practice gratitude. Journaling daily about events and difficulties was incredibly helpful in learning to love and understand myself.

At first I found it difficult to do what my therapist asked me, to write down positive things, but after several days it became much easier. Once I surrendered myself to God's purpose for me, my life changed completely. I started to notice how much I had to be grateful for. God had given me the husband of my dreams, children who love me deeply, and a house in the country complete with the pond I'd always wanted. Yet happiness eluded me. It wasn't until I took inventory of my life that I appreciated it. I started to take notice of the little things. A beautiful flower, the smell of rain, the feel of grass beneath my feet as I ground myself in the morning. There was an overwhelming amount of things to be grateful for. I started realizing that God was granting my requests and yet I never even noticed it! He began opening doors and bringing the right people into my life as only He can. I now have confidence in my ability to help others. I live with gratitude and love for my life today. That's something I never dreamed was in the cards for me. Gratitude made it possible.

Other things that have helped me to love myself is figuring out what makes me happy. Sounds simple, but I learned that material things will never bring me lasting joy. Money doesn't bring happiness. I know plenty of people with money who are miserable. I learned through watching my father that fame doesn't bring one joy either. Once his fame was over, depression and lack of purpose ruined his life. He drank and smoked himself into an early grave. I don't believe power brings happiness either unless it is being used to help others. Just look at our political figures. They don't represent any kind of happiness that I am looking for. It doesn't matter which party, none of them seem happy to me. I finally shut off the TV and opened my Bible. Too much negativity throws me out of alignment with God. Fear and negativity abound, keeping people stressed and worried. God wants us to be happy. We have nothing to fear regardless of the world's chaos. I make the choice daily to be happy and to look for the good around me. I notice a smile from strangers or the way the sun's rays come through the clouds. It's the simple things in life for me anymore. I live in awe of God's creations. I appreciate the details that he put into each and every thing. Nothing is insignificant.

I became aware of holistic remedies to help my body heal itself. I started to get off the prescription meds and replaced them with holistic herbs and teas. My brain fog cleared. I started to feel differently. I started to feel healthy – at last. My energy and stamina finally returned. I feel like a child again. My eyes are open to the beauty around me. I desire to learn and grow. My sleep has been restored. I pay attention now if something feels off. I understand that it is imperative to experience some discomfort in life; my life was once so painful that I prayed for God to bring an end to it. It was through surrendering my will and embracing God's will that I came to understand this lesson.

I have gained wisdom in my journey. I've learned the importance of setting goals and taking steps each day to achieve those goals. Proudly, I can now hold myself accountable for my life. There's no shame in finding someone to hold you accountable to begin. I am grateful to those people who helped hold me accountable during this time in my life. I was never taught the importance of chasing your dreams. Sadly people surrender in defeat, allowing the setbacks to terminate their pursuit of goals. This journey has proven my resilience to me. I see the strength that is the result of difficulties I endured. I joke with myself about the bad-ass I have become!

The truth is I don't really relate to who I was back then. I love who I am becoming. I no longer worry what others think of me. It's irrelevant to me these days. God has opened my eyes and shown me why I am needed. That's my focus. Helping others keeps me out of my head. It provides them a valuable service as well. It's a win-win situation perfectly created by God's design. I simply had to surrender my will and replace it with HIS.

Now loving myself, I maintain it with a daily routine. It keeps me feeling my very best.

I start with getting enough sleep. Something that had eluded me for years. Sleep is imperative for our bodies to recover and repair themselves. Be sure to get enough sleep daily.

I wake at a regular time each day. I enjoy a warm mushroom blend beverage for focus and energy.

I practice gratitude and daily devotion to God. Meditation is helpful for some. I find it difficult at times to stop the deluge of thoughts that fill my mind. I still practice as I've learned how beneficial it is for the mind and body connection. I will continue to practice and grow.

Exercise is crucial for my physical and mental health. I notice that after a period of inactivity that it is very difficult to get in the rhythm of an exercise routine. At almost 300 pounds it was a struggle to move. I had to start out slowly. Injuries were common as a result of my long term Prednisone use for a medical condition. Muscle tears and pulls insured a slow pace. Very slow. It's been over five years since I took off 80 pounds. I discovered how much I missed dancing. I treasure memories of me growing up in Scottsdale dancing with my neighbors. Remembering those times always brings a smile to me. Today I enjoy somatic and ecstatic dancing as my favorite ways to exercise. Hiking and swimming bring me joy as well. I encourage you to find something that brings you pleasure and incorporate it into your daily routine. It will help you become more likely to achieve your goals if it's something you enjoy.

Self care is a must. When I was depressed and sick, self care wasn't a priority for me. I had lost a lot of teeth because of neglect and a paralyzing fear of dentists. I finally found a lovely dentist who helped me through this fear with her compassion and empathy. She restored my smile. I can't contain my smile anymore! It feels amazing!

My skin was dry and my hair was brittle. It was in need of some intense care. I developed a skin care ritual focusing on cleansing, toning, and moisturizing using holistic ingredients. People commented that I was glowing. That definitely inspired me to continue. I'd struggled with the HS skin disorder. I quit smoking and eating a lot of processed foods and that resolved most of the problems stemming from the disorder. I started doing Epsom salt baths. That is also beneficial. I discovered the soaks help relieve others issues also. The magnesium in the Epsom salt helps immensely with my restless leg syndrome. I no longer take drugs like Lyrica or Gabapentin. I realize that when I experience pain or symptoms of illness that it's my body in need of rest. I give myself Grace as God has taught me to do.

I eat healthy food these days and limit my intake of processed food. I researched our food supply and became aware of everything I was putting into my body. I learned how major food companies have modified our food to keep us fat and addicted; they are spraying crops with cancer-causing chemicals to stop crop loss from bugs. This wasn't done in the consumers interest, but for profit. People are sicker than ever. Cancer, Alzheimer's, ADHD, and Autism are all skyrocketing. Big Pharma is banking on this continuing as their profits have never been higher. I believe God took me on this journey to increase my awareness about what is happening on this planet. To be aware and make the changes necessary. To tell others my story of navigating our medical system which was designed for profit, not healing. I wish to help others advocate for better treatment. I want to advocate for us to be given choices of how to proceed with our healthcare. I think people should be told about holistic therapies versus prescription drugs and nasty side effects. God wants us to be happy and healthy. If we get our gut health fixed then we should not only survive but thrive and help others do the same.

Psalms 73:26
My body and my heart may fail,
But God is the rock of my heart and my portion forever.

This year I am looking forward to growing an abundant, organic vegetable crop. Bryon and I have always had a small garden, but this is going to be a much bigger undertaking. I plan on making teas and tinctures to continue healing. I also plan on doing more canning and freezing then we have done in the past. I will prepare my home to become more self-sustaining in an attempt to eventually live off the grid. I will share my bounty with my friends and neighbors as God instructed me to do. It's my purpose. I am gratefully obedient to God the Father. He brought me back from the grave to fulfill this purpose. This is what fills my heart with joy and hope for the future. It is my reason for living these days. I encourage each of you to find out what matters most to you, to follow your heart and see where it leads you. Every day when I awake I welcome all of God's goodness into my life. Every day I am amazed at what transpires. Believe in yourself. Allow God to lead you. You will understand how important each of us is. We are each uniquely designed in His image. He has a specific reason for each of us. Through His Love of us, no one can harm us again. It doesn't mean we don't have problems. It means they can't hurt us and that it will pass. Lean on your beliefs for strength. Our difficulties bring us closer to God. Without those difficulties we wouldn't appreciate the good. Remember to practice gratitude for your blessings and the lessons and in this you will learn to love yourself.

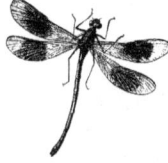

Move Forward

My faith has helped me to survive.
I owe everything to God just to be alive.

I am not as strong as I may look.
I owe my strength to everything I am learning from "The Book."

God created me with a specific purpose; I know he had a plan.
I don't care what others think, they can't possibly understand.

My reality changed when I surrendered to our Lord.
For it's only with His Guidance that I'm able to move forward.

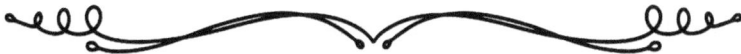

Routine

I developed a daily routine on my healing journey. I found that I needed structure in my life. Each morning I start my day with a gratitude practice. I thank God for giving me another day. I journal as I listen to a daily devotional/motivational video to focus on positive things each day. I drink mushroom coffee and take several supplements that help keep me feeling my best. I stretch and exercise my body. Not only does it help me stay fit but it is crucial for my mental health. It's rekindled my love of music and dancing. Ecstatic dancing is super easy and fun. No rules, just feel the music and move your body. I have noticed a difference on days that I am unable to exercise due to injury or time constraints. My mood tends to become more edgy and gloomy.

I practice breathwork and meditation to practice mindfulness. I have attended retreats to learn some techniques. It is a great way to meet like minded individuals! I always feel energized and reborn after breathwork sessions. You may also find videos on the internet. There are other ways of releasing energy like EFT or tapping. Whatever works best for you, do it.

Some people enjoy nature hikes, being near bodies of water or forest bathing to be beneficial as well. There is definitely something about being in nature that is healing. Take time to notice everything around you. The way the sun comes through the trees, the mushrooms attached to fallen logs, or the singing of birds. I am in awe of God's creations every time I am out in nature. Beauty abounds everywhere.

Self care routines are critical. During my worst bouts of depression I didn't care about taking care of myself. I struggled to brush my teeth some days. Thankfully I found a wonderful dentist who managed to save the teeth I have left. I quit coloring my hair. I have other things I'd rather do with my free time. Daily I moisturize my skin and face. I am embracing aging gracefully. When I was struggling with mental health issues, self care was never a priority. It became difficult for me to love myself. I gained a lot of weight and avoided looking in a mirror for years. I didn't love myself. I have forgiven myself for my imperfections. I am grateful for my body today. I am amazed at everything I have survived. I now love who I am becoming. I have realized that I am a good person. I am worthy of living a good life! When I was at my lowest point in life I prayed to God for guidance. He revealed my purpose is to help others. It fills my heart and soul with love. I wake each morning eager to start my day. Helping seniors and people with disabilities keeps me out of my head. It is so rewarding for me to help others. When I discovered my purpose my depression lifted. My heart literally filled with joy by being of service to others. As a bonus I have made some wonderful new friends. They helped to fill the void in my life from deaths in my family.

As a person who struggled with body dysmorphia for most of my life, writing down three things I like about myself was challenging at first. I was so caught up in trying to be perfect I hated this 300 pound person staring at me in the mirror. I had to break it down into baby steps. Others saw beauty in me that I failed to see. Instead focusing on physical beauty I dove inward. I discovered a kind, caring, wounded child who just needed to be loved.

I had always thought of myself as a good friend to people. I always helped others when I could.

I connected with animals and they trusted me. I discovered that I was capable of feeling/sensing others' energy. Through my journaling I realized I had resilience and strength. I discovered that I matter. Shockingly, journaling proved to me how fleeting time is. Recently I discovered a journal I had written 20 years ago. Eerily I was struggling with the same issues I was dealing with now. I languished my life away waiting for someone to come rescue me from me. Waiting for some doctor to fix me. Surely the next pill will cure me. It wasn't happening.

Journaling these days holds me accountable. It's also a great way to remember things. It's especially helpful for me with my brain injury. I make it fun. I have all kinds of stickers. Different gel pens to mix things up. Don't complicate it. Do it messy. Don't overthink it. Write whatever comes naturally. Get out your negativity on paper. Release your worries to the universe. Then practice gratitude for the blessings each day. You will be surprised how your life will change.

I have started eating healthy. Eliminating processed foods wasn't easy, but was so beneficial. I have less pain and inflammation in my body. I am eating grass fed beef and organic free range chicken whenever possible. My family is loving all the changes as they, too, are experiencing the benefits.

I was never taught the importance of having a routine or holding myself accountable. During my journey I discovered that my life had gotten out of control because I had never set any goals. I never had a plan of action. By holding myself accountable I am achieving my goals and dreams. I no longer languish in depression and remorse. I have forgiven myself because I didn't know any better. Through loving myself I see how competent I am. I now understand the importance of self care. I discovered how much I love dancing again. It frees my soul. I spent years worrying what others thought of me. These days I don't give it a second thought. I no longer live with fear or feelings of unworthiness. I know my worth! I dance whenever the music moves me. It's not uncommon these days to find me doing ecstatic dancing out in my pool.

I refuse to give up on myself. On the less than perfect days I give myself grace. I value serenity more than others' opinions. I have learned it's all about balance. Give and take. Yin and yang. I've embraced the high and the lows. I live fully in the present. God has already gifted me with over 20 bonus years. Each night before bed I journal about my day. I thank God for the gift of another day, smiling knowing He is with me always.

It can be difficult to begin a routine, but not impossible. To start you need to have a goal and from there you take teeny tiny steps until you achieve it. I would set huge goals and then become so intimidated that I was defeated before ever beginning. I needed to get my ego in check. My fear of failure kept me stuck for years. I needed someone to hold me accountable. I didn't care enough about myself to just do it alone. I would constantly fail. I asked a friend to join me in exercising. She found it necessary to have an accountability partner as well. Once you find a buddy you need to set a date to begin. You must stick to the schedule. You can't disappoint your friend after all. Commit and follow through. Live your life with integrity. Stay true to your word. There are guaranteed to be days that you aren't feeling it. No excuses. Do it anyway. After around 90 days you will notice a big difference. You will see results of your hard work. You will have initiated your routine! Whether you want to lose weight, quit drinking, or learn something new, the first step is always the hardest. I promise that stepping out of your comfort zone, while challenging, offers huge rewards. I've learned that it's what makes us grow. Setting goals, taking baby steps towards those goals, and finally completing your list of goals is the true purpose of life. We are constantly changing, growing, and learning new things. Life is an amazing gift. Surviving difficulty enables you to grow and help others through similar situations. It brings us together with the purpose of community. We are here for a reason. Each of our unique experiences make us who we are. We must share our struggles by telling our stories. We must normalize having difficult days without shame. We must learn to endure discomfort because it teaches us valuable lessons. Finally we come together to support each other.

Our country has become so divided. We have lost ourselves in search of wealth, fame, and power.

We must take ownership of ourselves and our shortcomings. We must stop being victims of life. For years I blamed my unhappiness on things that had happened to me. Things others had done to me kept me feeling broken and unworthy, but this was only because I had allowed myself to feel this way. I kept waiting for doctors to find a cause for all my illnesses, believing the next pill would fix my life. It wasn't until I realized that nobody was coming to save me that I was able to take back control over my life. I had attempted to become sober several times. I truly thought I wanted sobriety at the time, but I would always relapse. I found myself reflecting on things from the past and blaming people for hurting or disappointing me, leading me to relapse. I had to take ownership for my shortcomings and recognize that what I was really doing was using it as an excuse to relapse. ("Well, if you knew my story, you'd drink too" mentality.) I now understand it was my brain trying to rationalize having a drink, not an actual reason to pick up again. We need to stop pointing fingers at others and acknowledge and heal our own baggage. Leave the victim mentality for others. It no longer serves who you are becoming through your routine. You must be completely honest with yourself and acknowledge that you are the reason for your current situation. Once you recognize the problem then you may make the necessary changes to remedy the situation. One routine at a time.

Taking ownership of our shortcomings is not an easy endeavor. You have to step away from victimhood and into ownership of your life. It is a painful but necessary process. Checking the beliefs that you've been raised with is difficult. Cultural beliefs are instilled in us since childhood. They become ingrained into our daily lives. We must be honest with ourselves and identify the things that are no longer relevant in our life. Only then do we grow and heal. I am now open to new things and experiences to broaden my mind. I treat each day as a blessing. I am eager to see what each day brings. I spent decades watching TV to kill time. It was such a colossal waste of my life. That waste of time would be my one regret.

We should be mindful about life. Practicing gratitude has profound effects. Gratitude reminds us of how far we have come. Gratitude practice also proves that life isn't as bad as we believe it to be. Once I began practicing an attitude of gratitude my life changed immensely. I realized that I already had everything I wanted. The problem was that I didn't appreciate all that I had. It was eye opening. I started to notice the little things that brought me joy. Bees pollinating flowers, birds singing, holding hands with Bryon, smiles from a stranger. Everything seemed to be a blessing. I began to feel worthy of love. I began to radiate love and joy. All things that had eluded me my entire life. God showed me my purpose. I thank Him each morning for the gift of another day.

I set new goals immediately after completing each one. It's a continuing cycle of finding one's purpose: following a routine, and practicing gratitude. Today it is easier for me. I'm a work in progress. While challenging to change there's no better feeling than when you own your life. The good, the bad, and everything in between – it's what makes us human.

So give yourself grace and get busy creating a routine for yourself. You are worthy! The only thing stopping you is you. I believe in you, you should too! You are a unique individual designed by God. Lean on Him during your tough times and praise Him during the bountiful times. We make this life way harder than it needs to be. God made it simple. Follow the Golden Rule. Lead with Love and you're guaranteed to find happiness. If you see someone struggling, help when you can. Practice kindness to others and remember to be kind to yourself as well. Remember that everyone is going through something that you have no knowledge of. Developing a routine will help you to change your life. I challenge you to prove me wrong. Make yourself a priority. Get plenty of rest, eat healthy, and take small steps each day to achieve your goals. Push through any ego and self doubt. I believe in you.

Make the decision to change the things you know deep down that you must change. Then help those close to you to do the same when they are ready. What a beautiful world it would be if everyone learned to love themselves in this way. It could happen. With God's love for us, I believe anything is possible.

Hebrews 10:24-25
And let us consider how to stir up one another to love and good works, not neglecting to meet together, as is the habit of some, but encouraging one another, and all the more as you see the Day drawing near.

My Routine

Discipline is something I was never taught and has turned out to be so important in my healing. I'm sharing my daily routine to inspire you to make your own routine to heal yourself and find self love.

- practice gratitude everyday.
- serve others with kindness
- wake early
- prepare mushroom coffee
- take my supplements
- wash face, brush teeth, and moisturize
- dance or walking workout
- set goals
- step out of comfort zone/ challenge myself
- maintain my friendships
- rest and recharge
- communicate feelings/ storytelling
- therapy – to manage PTSD and panic attacks
- meditation
- adequate restful sleep
- journal/write poems
- get out in nature
- notice the small things
- listen to music
- make healthy meals and eat with my family
- walk in the woods
- have a bonfire
- dream about the future
- forgive myself for past mistakes
- country drives
- stay out of my own head
- daily devotional
- pray to maintain alignment with God
- live in the present

Forgiveness

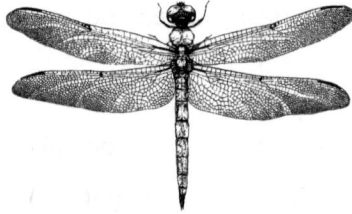

Forgiveness has been a difficult process for me. Being abused as a child left a lasting impression on me. For the longest time I prayed for vengeance on those who had harmed me. I wanted karma to make them suffer. I used alcohol as an anger suppressant. I wanted to be numb. Rage lies just below the surface at all times. As a sober person these days drinking is no longer an option for me. I had to find a way to deal with the flood of emotions that surfaced with my sobriety. These days I gladly give my worries to God. It is the only thing that I have found to restore my sense of peace.

In life when relationships end or people die there is usually a sense of closure of some kind. I needed closure for a lot of things, but was never able to get it. As a child I confronted Don, because I needed my grandma to believe me. Unfortunately that never happened. Instead she trusted my molester over me. I felt betrayed by the one woman I knew loved me. It cut me deep in my core. I loved my grandma and I had to forgive her for never hearing my pain.

My mother was another person I had to forgive. I now understand her struggles with alcohol and gambling addiction. I now know that she was trying to escape from something, too. I will never forget the things she did to me, but I had to forgive. Not for her sake, but for my own. For way too many years I blamed my mother for all the wrongs in my life. These days I understand that I am ultimately the one responsible for myself. Determined not to hurt people as she did, I do my best to be kind to others. I don't linger on the negativity from my past, but I focus on becoming a better, more loving and empathetic person each day. Forgiveness made it all possible.

I have forgiven all the men in my life who have ever hurt me. I now appreciate the lessons I learned from them. Adrian taught me about betrayal, John taught me about resilience, and Charles made me see that there is real evil in this world. My father showed me that not all dads are fathers. Fathers are supposed to protect their children. I understand that my dad did the best he could, I forgive him. I now know that hurt people hurt people. Forgiving them was necessary for closure.

Today my relationship with God has opened my eyes to see that without forgiveness I was the one to suffer. I held the pain caused by others deep inside of me for way too long. Replaying the bad memories repeatedly kept me languishing with loneliness. It kept me from healing and growing. The only solution was to forgive those people for the things that I felt were unforgivable. It became clear to me when I began to understand Jesus' ultimate sacrifice for us when he was crucified on the cross for our sins. If he was able to forgive, then certainly I needed to let go of my pain and anger as well. Immediately after praying for those I forgave, my peace was restored. Forgiveness made it possible.

> *Immediately after praying for those I forgave, my peace was restored. Forgiveness made it possible.*

As an exercise in forgiveness, I wrote a letter to my mom. I encourage you to do the same to help you process and let go. Letter to Mom is a little long, as there was a lot to say...

Forgiveness - Letter to Mom

Dear Mom,

It's been 16 years since you've been gone. The grief I still feel is immense. There is a huge part of my heart that will always be empty. I will never forget finding you 12 days before Christmas. Or myself rifling through your cupboards in search of alcohol to numb the pain. I was dumbfounded when there wasn't a drop in the house. I wasn't prepared for that day. I guess one never really is. I was really enjoying the time we had together. Things were finally good between us. You had gotten to know my family. You fell in love with Bryon and the boys. Remember you were so mad when I married him? You refused to come to my wedding, even though we offered to pay for your and Dad's flight. My wedding day was perfect except for the fact that you two were missing. Our friends allowed us the use of their beautiful country estate. Another friend dumped confetti out of his small plane above the event. Bryon's brother cooked a 46 pound salmon and the rest of our friends brought dishes to pass. We combined our wedding and our baby shower. The night ended with everyone celebrating around a large bonfire. A justice of the peace provided the service; complete with the playing of the song The Rose. I, of course, was overwhelmed with everything being eight months pregnant. I fought through tears during the entire service.

My mother-in-law Lila approached me after the service and questioned my tears during the ceremony. She mumbled something about that if I was so unhappy I shouldn't have gone through with marrying her son.

Brody was born a month later. I was so in love with him. He was a dream come true for me. The product of the union of Bryon and I. It was amazing. Bryon would frequently get up with me at night and watch as I breastfed Brody. I finally had the family of my dreams. Suddenly however, things changed. I developed Postpartum depression. I couldn't stop crying. I was placed on antidepressants again. I had to stop breastfeeding and I hit the bottle again. Alcohol was my coping method. I enjoyed being a stay-at-home mom, but I got lonely. My friends' kids were teenagers or fully grown. They didn't want to hang out with me and the baby.

Bryon's 40th birthday came and I had organized a surprise party for him at a local tavern. All our friends and family came to celebrate. Someone asked Bryon how he enjoyed being a daddy again. He mentioned we were thinking of having another. That's when my mother-in-law shoved a handful of condoms into Bryon's pocket in front of our friends. We didn't know I was already pregnant at the time. We found out two weeks later that Jake was on the way.

When raising my boys I often thought of my childhood. I thought about sending them away for three months every year as you had done with us. I could have never been away from them that long. I also couldn't imagine dumping my six-week-old child on anyone, much less my mother! Your explanation that you did it out of concern for your grieving mother's wellbeing was far from convincing. You never did anything for anyone but yourself.

I have been on a healing journey lately. I'm about to celebrate six years off cigarettes and alcohol. I changed my diet and started dancing again. I have managed to lose 80 lbs. I have learned the importance of being self disciplined. Most people learn these things from their parents, unfortunately I was never enlightened by either of you.

I am getting healthier every day. I am no longer taking a bucketful of meds. I am doing things holistically. I even have a little greenhouse. I plan to grow flowers, herbs, and vegetables to try and stay healthy. It will become a medicinal garden to continue on my healing journey.

I have also undergone a spiritual awakening. Losing Dad, Grandma six months later, and then you the following year literally broke me. The pain from grief was overwhelming. I crawled inside the bottle of rum and literally tried to drown myself drinking a handle of rum every three days for several years on end.

Before Grandma died I promised her that I would help Tracy someday. Do you remember the nasty fight between you and Tracy following grandma's funeral? When I gave Tracy my Oldsmobile '98 and sent her back to Georgia? Five weeks later she ended up getting arrested smuggling drugs after returning to Georgia. She did about a year in jail for that from what I remember. Once she got out she begged me to help her get her act together.

I welcomed her into our home. She set up residence in our computer room. I didn't allow her to drink while she lived with us. I helped her through detoxing. She slept for hours and raided the kitchen at night. It went on for weeks, then months. Finally I insisted she get a job. She started working in the next town over. I took her to work and picked her up daily. It was going great. She was very hopeful. I found her an apartment close to her job. I furnished the apartment with furniture that we found online. Bryon and I would run all over Wisconsin to pick up free furniture for her new place. Finally, the day came and we moved her in. She was so grateful. We even got her a bike to ride to work.

She got paid the day we dropped the bike off. After we left she hopped on the bike attempting to pedal up an incredibly steep hill to the liquor store and wiped out, dislocating her shoulder and making her unable to work. I was livid. So much time and effort wasted. I promised: never again.

I contacted her landlord and thankfully they allowed her out of the rental contract. I bought her a bus ticket back to Georgia. We talked daily on the phone but I could tell she wasn't doing well. After a couple years apart I received a call from a hospital saying that her organs had begun shutting down. They needed a signature from a family member allowing them to disconnect her from life support.

I hopped on a flight to Mississippi and met with my friend Jerome who drove me up to Georgia. At the hospital I was greeted by her latest boyfriend. He assured me that when she got released he would never let her drink again. He honestly thought she was going to get out of the hospital?!

The nurse took me into another room where I signed the papers. They told me Tracy's brain was toxic. Tracy had no idea of what was happening. She was restrained and tied to the bed. Tubes were everywhere. She thrashed around and screamed incoherently. I couldn't hold back the tears knowing I would never see her again. Neither would either of her children. What have I done? I returned home to Bryon and the boys. I thought about her children. I prayed they would forgive me for what I felt I had to do.

Once home the reality of the situation hit hard when her cremated remains were delivered. I felt so incredibly alone. The pain of grief had been resurrected. It took over my life. Back in the bottle for a couple more years. The mental anguish forced me to dissociate from the world. I languished in my room for the next two years.

My friend Jimmy had come to visit. We stopped at the local cheese store. I wanted to give him some squeaky cheese curds fresh from the factory! As I rushed into the store my foot caught the rug's edge and I fell to the ground. I did not want to ruin Jimmy's visit. We went to breakfast and then he returned to Illinois. After he departed I told Bryon I thought I might have broken something and he took me to the ER. They x-rayed my neck since I had gotten lodged up against the door. Turns out that I fractured my elbow and ankle and sprained my wrist. In the x-ray they spotted nodules throughout my lungs. A CT scan of my lungs was ordered which uncovered a mass in my liver. Then I developed PMR. It affected every joint in my body. I felt like an eighty year old woman. The doctors prescribed me Prednisone. Within months I blew up to 300 pounds. I hated everything about myself and my life.

My depression was at its worst. I did not want to live any longer. I couldn't kill myself though. I was angry at God. If there was a God then I challenged Him to take me out of this world. I questioned why he had spared my life years ago when I had a cardiac arrest. Why did he spare me? I wanted to understand.

Exhausted, physically and spiritually ill, I surrendered my life to God. God you take the reins, I give my life to you. Show me the way. He showed me that life isn't meant to be difficult. That we make things difficult. He showed me that happiness is not the opposite of depression. The cure for depression is purpose. God revealed my purpose of friendship and love. To achieve this happiness I had to forgive those who wronged me. I needed to accept that sometimes we never get apologies or closure. So many times I asked myself: "How could such a beautiful woman be such a monster?" I had to let that question go. Mom, I had to forgive you. I'm writing this today to do just that.

I forgive you for leaving me with Grandma at six weeks old after your father died. I have tried to imagine how you could hand me off as such a tiny baby. It wouldn't have been possible for me to leave my kids with anyone at that tender age.

I forgive you for leaving us in the care of people who hurt me/us. I know you and Dad were quite the socialites in the early 70s, but things happened while you were otherwise engaged. Being locked in a closet by a sitter and made to do unimaginable things while threatened not to tell anyone at ages three and four.

I forgive you for letting friends and neighbors look after us while growing up. I am now grateful for those people who actually cared for us like the Brendles and the Lombardos. They helped me to believe loving caring families actually existed.

I forgive you for letting my dog Benji "escape" when I went to my first sleepover after we moved to Vegas. I never believed your story about him getting out under the fence. It only made me doubt you more. I know you sold him.

I forgive you for selling my horse Dandy without any warning. My beautiful baby girl. My dream horse. My confidant and best friend. I remember the many hours we spent together. Our bond was special. We were going to be together forever. Maybe ride the rodeo circuit? Or get her to Wisconsin on the farm?

Those dreams all shattered that day. We started at the Fashion Show Mall. You were offering to buy me anything. I was incredibly suspicious when I noticed you checking your watch. I remember the phone call upon our return home. You ordered me to get ready to go to the ranch where she was boarded. There I noticed a trailer backing up and thought we were getting a new boarder at the ranch. I couldn't have been more wrong when the man got out of his truck and handed you a check for Dandy.

To say that I had been blindsided is an understatement. I was devastated and Dandy was terrified. She had never been trailered alone. I remember I was crying hysterically when I left for home on foot. I hyperventilated and was struggling to breathe. I saw Kenny out in the desert with his falcon. He noticed me crying and waved me over. I explained what happened. He lit up and handed me a joint. That was the first time I'd ever experimented with drugs. You broke your end of the deal. So I broke my promise and dove head first into the drug and partying scene.

I forgive you for cashing the check for my horse and dragging me to the casino while you lost every last dollar from her sale. That was the beginning of my hating you. I began to hate everyone. I hated myself the most for not saving Dandy.

I forgive you for not getting me any help after I was molested by Don, a family friend, at Tracy's 9th birthday party. I was only 9 at the time. Grandma didn't believe me and made me confront him in front of his wife the following day. They labeled me a liar and a filthy minded little girl. Isn't that crazy? You were told but did nothing. No one got me any help afterwards either. I was a child who needed love and understanding, yet I was treated as if nothing happened and branded a liar.

I forgive you for losing several homes and destroying friendships with people I had grown close to because of your compulsive gambling.

I forgive you for years of mental and emotional torture. Hurt people hurt people right?

I forgive you for using me to get money for you. What did you make from setting me up on those dates with those businessmen when I was 17? I sincerely hope it was worth it to you cause it cost me any self esteem I might have had for myself. Only now do I understand my true worth. 50 years of self loathing was plenty.

I forgive you for forcing us into modeling as children. I developed severe body dysmorphia as a result. I started binging/purging and using laxatives to lose weight. I eventually developed a hole in my stomach from the laxatives and required medication to coat my stomach lining so it could heal. I also overdosed several times using speed to control my appetite throughout high school. I was so desperate for your approval. I wanted to make you proud of me.

I forgive you for never attending my horse show. I only had one and you missed it by attending an Old-Timers game in New York.

I forgive you for not attending my wedding or contributing in any way. At least it was drama free.

I forgive you for missing the births of my children. Their births were private and intimate between me and Bryon. Again, no drama without you there.

I forgive you for not visiting me or helping me after my cardiac arrest. I told myself you didn't realize that I was actually brought back from death. Bryon breathed for me when I was blue lipped and lifeless until I could be defibrillated by the EMTs.

I forgive you for not being there when I needed help with taking care of Grandma, raising two young boys, and recovering from a near death experience.

I forgive you for betraying and stealing from relatives and longtime friends. The amount of wire transfers I found after your death blew my mind. Wow! That was quite the addiction you had going there.

I forgive you for sending me back to John after you knew he broke my nose by headbanging me during a fight. You should have protected me, but you never did. You knew that he was a controlling coke addict and alcoholic. Yet you told me to work it out. You thought that he was a great catch and that I was being dramatic. Again no one ever believed me. It conditioned me to believe that I didn't matter. It made me feel unworthy of love.

I forgive you for forcing me to get an abortion or you would put me out into the streets. I'm sure you were only looking out for me right? You didn't want me to experience the pain of putting a child up for adoption like you did right? I pray for God's forgiveness everyday for what I did.

I forgive you for not getting me help afterwards when I became despondent.

I forgive you for throwing me out of the house when I finally began seeing someone who made me laugh, enter Charles. I married him 10 days after we met. The biggest mistake of my life. Forced me to grow up and face some of the scariest times of my life over the next six months. I own that. It was my choice. I accepted the repercussions of that decision. I am now getting the therapy needed for everything he put me through. My desire to get back at you left me with severe PTSD.

I forgive you for what I believe was a mercy killing of Grandma, your own mother. Although I understand someone fantasizing about hurting their mother, I believe you may have crossed the line. Something wasn't quite as you described her final night. I felt your deception through my whole body. I'm sure the hospice nurse felt it too. May God forgive you.

Regardless I now see that all of it needed to happen. I forgive it all. It's made my life today possible. Without everything I would never have ended up here today. Happily married with two beautiful boys and a bonus son!

I owe my life today to God. It's only through His grace that I am here today. I believe I have gone through these challenges to help strengthen me for my life today. God has given me everything I asked for. He gave me what you never could. I had to let go of the past and forgive before I could appreciate my life. I practice gratitude daily. I am serving a life of purpose. Helping seniors and people with disabilities live independently in their homes. Years of caregiving definitely prepared me for this role. I love my clients. They have become like family to me and helped fill the void. I struggled with grief for a long time. Losing my family has reminded me of how fleeting time is. I treasure my life today. So grateful to have been given these past 21 bonus years.

I miss you mom. I forgive you. I truly did love you.

Psalm 130:4
For with you there is true forgiveness,
So that you may be held in awe.

The exercise continues... I was going to write a letter to my dad, but I barely knew him and I'll never know WHY was he unable to love us. If your parents are still alive, get their stories. Try to have some understanding. And share your experiences with your own children. Know each other more. Understanding brings forgiveness.

Forgiveness - Letter to Men

I guess the first man I must forgive is my father. He was more like a stranger to me actually than a father. Many people admired him for his athletic prowess. I do remember growing up at the ballpark. Eating hot dogs and cracker jacks. I loved being at the ball games. I loved the atmosphere of the ballpark. The sights and sounds. The vendors yelling out their products for purchase. The crack of the ball when the bat hit it. I loved watching him pitch. I was so proud that he was my father. After the game we would meet him under the stadium where he would be busy signing autographs. He would scoop us up in his arms. People were always commenting on his beautiful family. He was my hero when I was young.

After he retired from playing ball things changed rapidly. He drank more and more with each year. Smoked cigarettes like a chimney. He held various jobs. Car salesman, prison guard, owned a car radio business, and finally drove a school bus for disabled children. He was a very honest man. I was taught by him at an early age about the importance of honesty. Lying got us an immediate whooping.

He never became involved or interested in my life. He was never a part of any of the important things in my life. He wasn't available for my wedding or the birth of my children. In fact I remember him telling me I should elope when I found the right husband. My dad promised that he would give me the money that it would have cost for the event as my wedding gift. He never gave me a penny for my wedding to Bryon. They didn't attend my wedding even though I offered to purchase the plane tickets. I was never a priority for him. Even when he learned about some of the things I endured as a child, he never spoke to me about any of it. He acted like he didn't know. I could never count on him to protect me.

My dad was very easy going most of the time. My mother challenged him constantly. Her lies and deception went against everything he claimed to stand for. I only saw him lose his cool a couple of times. Once punching a hole through a hollow core door instead of hitting my mother, even though at the time I wouldn't have blamed him if he did. She literally broke him financially, emotionally, and otherwise.

My hero became a functioning alcoholic. He was chronically sick with lung issues yet he smoked two packs of unfiltered Camel cigarettes daily. He would work and then come home at night and drink his scotch and water until he passed out. He would smoke his cigarettes outside and then come inside and do his nebulizer and breathing treatments. When I asked him why he kept smoking even though he couldn't breathe, his reply was it was the only thing that brought him happiness. He wanted to die. He became a shell of the once good looking, athletic man I had admired as a child.

I forgive my father for never being there for me. For never protecting me. I never knew why he couldn't be a father to me.

Why did he allow things with my mother to get so bad? Why was I so unlovable to him?

I never knew the story of his upbringing. I know his father died when he was young. I never understood how he could have walked away from his kids from his first marriage. He always said he didn't want to confuse them. He managed to fulfill his financial duties, but that was it. I feel like that is why he never connected with me and Tracy. From the outside we were a happy, perfect family. Our real home life was a tragedy. I yearned for love. I started dating older men I think in some attempt to make up for the lack of a father figure.

I forgive my father for being unable to be there for me. It forced me to realize that love has to come from within. My whole life I was in search of love. Fifty plus years later I now understand that the love I needed was from myself and not from him after all. Sorry Dad that we never really got to know each other. I am grateful that Brody had some memories with his grandfather before you died. Thank you for taking us around Vegas before you died. Brody had a great time. I was grateful for the time that we spent together. I love you. I hope you found your joy again.

The other man I wish to forgive is my husband. I forgive him for purely being a man. By just being a man I wanted him to pay for the others who had hurt me so deeply. I knew that by just being a man he wasn't capable of loving me as I had needed. He tried harder to love me though than any other person in my life. He cared enough to stand by me through all the difficulties, even when I pushed him away. He listened to me as I tried to understand myself.

He encouraged me to want to live again. His patience is never ending. I appreciate everything he has done for me over our years together.

I forgive him for refusing to fight with me when we first got together. I had grown to understand that men were only interested in me for one thing. Subconsciously I wanted to strike first. I was constantly waiting for the other shoe to drop early in our relationship. He seemed too good to be true. I would often instigate a fight between us just to see what he would do. I constantly needed validation from him that he wasn't going to leave me. Bryon's love never wavered. I challenged him to love me when I was unlovable. I forgive him for refusing to give up on me. Bryon knew my worth before I did. He became my hero where others had failed. Bryon never left my side when I got sick or I went into rehab. He breathed for me during my cardiac arrest. He became my memory after my brain injury. He took control and managed to run his business, tend to the children, and support me during my various illnesses. He never complained. He just did it. I am grateful to Bryon for everything he has done and continues to do for me. I had to kiss a lot of frogs before I found my prince charming. Our love is what I had been in search of my entire life. We recently celebrated thirty two years together. He was the stability that I had always longed for. He is my safe place to fall. I thank God for bringing us together. God knew what I needed all along. He knew I needed Bryon.

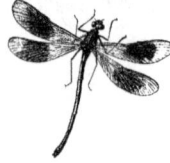

Life Today

Suddenly my load has lightened
I live with joy and am no longer frightened.

I look forward to each new day.
I begin with gratitude and remember to pray.

My life is a reminder of God's grace.
I love spreading joy all over the place.

Helping those who are lonely and depressed.
I help them out and show them that they are blessed.

Practicing gratitude has been life changing for me.
Jesus made it possible, I just had to believe.

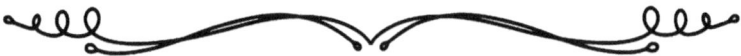

Healthy Relationships

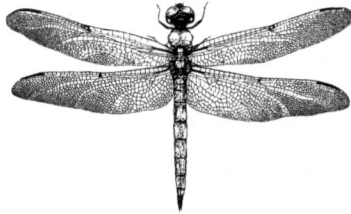

Boundaries

When one gets sober, boundaries must come into play to avoid relapse. Alcohol was my coping mechanism for most of my life. Chronic PTSD and depression issues often caused me to relapse. Dual diagnosis is a tricky thing. Being a highly sensitive person causes me to feel things deeply. I used alcohol to not feel. I no longer can reach for a drink to calm down or relax. Deeply buried feelings keep rising to the surface to be dealt with. Waves of strong emotions are hard to deal with especially when one is triggered. Boundaries are necessary because others don't always understand that their actions trigger you. Boundaries help others to understand what is expected and what things won't be tolerated.

It's all about balance. I understand that I had accepted behaviors from others that I could no longer tolerate. For instance Bryon would say things jokingly to me and I would take it personally. I no longer found the humor in it. His words unknowingly made me feel bad. I know that was never his intention. I had to speak up for myself and implement boundaries to eliminate the anger from what I perceived to be hurtful words. He resisted because I was making everything about me and he believed I was "too sensitive." He believed I was deliberately taking things the wrong way. At times it became a battle of wills. I was determined to enforce these boundaries as if my life depended on it, because it actually does. Never ever did I think my sobriety would destroy my marriage, but it caused us some time for reflection on if it was still right for us. We both refused to give up on each other. Today cooler heads prevail most of the time. Our love for each other was never in question, but we all had to adjust to the new me. Bryon is a gift from God. God gave me the strength to stick to my boundaries so I could heal. Together our love is stronger today after understanding the need for boundaries.

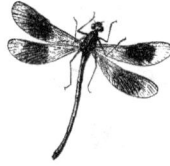

In the Zone

Do whatever it takes to stay in the zone.
This is especially true when you're feeling alone.

Do not sabotage yourself or your dreams.
Life isn't really as bad as it seems.

Do whatever it takes to stay in the zone.
Reach out and call a friend on the phone.

Stay focused and learn to believe in you.
You are important, you matter in all that you do.

Do whatever it takes to stay in the zone.
Remain calm and allow Jesus to lead you home.

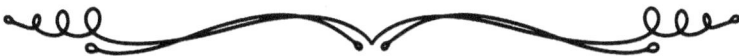

Bad experiences in past relationships is what ultimately taught me what I learned about how to have a good relationship.

Good Relationships

After a short but brutal marriage to Charles, I never wanted to be in a relationship again. The terror and violence inflicted by him left me doubting my judgment. He was the last of many bad relationships. I learned a lot because Charles was a complete psychopath. He lied to me about everything. He lied about his age and never told me that he was an ex convict until after we married. He had no remorse. I was just a tool he used to get what he wanted. He beat me so badly once that it hurt to breathe. My chest had different colors of bruises from brown to yellow and green. He held my precious dog hostage if I ever left his sight, he threatened to kill Max if I didn't return. My mind was constantly racing to figure a safe way out of the situation. I prayed for a hero.

Finally the opportunity arrived for my escape. Charles abandoned me and Max at a hotel in Florida. He took my car in the morning leaving Max and me in the motel. We were evicted because my credit card had been declined. Luckily the front desk clerk overheard me telling his mother I would call the police if my car was not returned. Thankfully he came back to the motel at 3 am and the clerk called the cops for me. I made my way back to Georgia and managed to pawn some jewelry to make it back to Wisconsin. Later I filed for and was granted an annulment.

After Charles was back in custody I was left to deal with the aftermath. The bills from being on the run with Charles had finally caught up to me. I didn't know what to do next. That's when Gale took me to Madison to meet with a lawyer about declaring bankruptcy and stopped at The Sandbar Sports Arena and I met Bryon. He seemed like such a sweet man. He had obviously been blindsided by his wife's departure. Starting a new relationship was the furthest thing from my mind at the time. However, Bryon and I couldn't deny our chemistry. We quickly became inseparable. He made me laugh. I could be vulnerable with him and I felt like he didn't judge me. We didn't dive into bed. Both of us were still legally married to other people. Neither of us wanted to fall in love, yet I believe God had other plans for us. It felt so natural. Bryon had all the qualities that I looked for in a man. Humorous, hard worker, independent, honest, and kind. He was an animal lover and had rescued many cats. He had a huge heart and wasn't afraid to show it. He had built himself a beautiful ranch home in the county. The crazy part was I drove past his house every year of my life on the way to my grandmother's farm. He was about 20 miles away from me all along.

I had always wanted a place in the country where I could have animals. I envisioned a pond and some acreage. I yearned for a man who loved me for me. I wanted someone who would give me the family I had always dreamed of. I needed someone to protect me from myself after going through the Charles ordeal.

God brought me my hero. Literally Bryon saved my life. He supported me repeatedly when I tried to get and stay sober. He was there when I had to check into a psychiatric hospital after a bad reaction to antidepressants. He stuck by me through numerous rehab stints. His love for me never wavered. He believed in me when I had lost all hope. He handled all responsibilities that I was unable to do during my recovery. He never complained. He is the love I yearned for all my life. When I practice gratitude, Bryon is on top of the list after God. Grateful for him staying with me through it all. I haven't been easy to deal with. I am a handful. Bryon is the capable and understanding lover and friend that I always needed. We complete one another. I am truly blessed to have him as my husband and best friend.

We have survived many things that could have destroyed our marriage. My health issues, having a child with a disability, my alcoholism, and my mental illness. Bryon's love was the glue that kept it together. He stood by me even when he didn't know how to help me. He attended almost all of my doctors appointments. He is my memory now for the things that I don't quite remember. He is the strongest, most patient person I have ever encountered. That isn't to say that we agree on everything, but we love each other enough to work things out.

No one in my life had ever given me the stability and empathy that Bryon has given to me. It seems strange that I have been with him now for more than half of my lifetime. I admire him intensely. He lives his life with integrity and passion. Our children are blessed to have such a loving father. I never experienced the kind of parental love Bryon has for his boys. Unconditional love and he is always there for them. I never had that in my life. I hope someday our children will understand how lucky they were to have him as their father. I look back on our life together now with so much love and gratitude.

My advice is to never give up on finding love. I believe there is someone for everyone. The secret is to know what you are looking for in someone and never settle for less. I believed God had me kiss a lot of frogs so that when I met Bryon I would appreciate him. I wasn't looking for love but God knew best when he brought us together. For that I will be forever grateful!

I am also grateful to God for removing certain people from my life. I realize that some people are only with us for a season in our life. I desperately tried to hold on to friendships out of some sense of loyalty. By doing so I allowed people to treat me horribly in an attempt to save the friendship. It always left me feeling empty and lost. I was ghosted by people who

I thought would be part of my life forever. It was a reality check long overdue. I did an inventory of my life and realized that I was on a totally different path than the person I once was. I no longer needed people who couldn't understand the metamorphosis that had transpired in my life. God filled the empty places in my heart with the right people now. I see the good that has come from the struggles. I see that during the solitude I had become a friend to myself. I started to love myself for the person I was becoming. God had filled my heart with grace and forgiveness. I forgave those who hurt me. I wish them well on their journey. Slowly new people came into my life and filled the void. My heart swelled up with love for others. I started making new friends with more like minded, empowered individuals. I have met some wonderful women with whom I can share my innermost thoughts and feelings. I don't fear judgment from these women either. It is so rewarding to have a tribe of girlfriends again! No more silly, competitive or backstabbing friends for me. God is truly working miracles. Together we can bring about the changes that we desperately need in life. I no longer fear being alone. I am a survivor.

Philippians 4:13
For all things I have the strength through the
one who gives me power.

God has helped me to love myself once and for all. Out of all the relationships in my life the relationship I had been in search of was my relationship with God. Through His love and Mercy I am now able to love myself. That has been huge in my recovery. It is only possible for that reason. By having self love I can love myself through difficult seasons these days. I refuse to surrender to the self talk that created so much havoc in my life.

These days I ask for discernment from God before making any changes in my life. God has gifted me with beautiful friends, clients, and job opportunities. My relationship with God will always be first and foremost. My love for myself must be next before I can love others. You can't pour from an empty cup as they say. These days I have an abundance of love for others. My days are filled with joy.

Relationships take work. Our lives are constantly changing. Friends may come and go. Those relationships that you want to endure require care and attention. It is too easy to get wrapped up in our daily routines that we allow our friendships to fall by the wayside. This is your reminder to tend to your friendships. They are what make our lives so unique and worthwhile. They are what make humans different from other species. We need to nurture those relationships that we value. Friends make our life worth living!

Look for the lessons in the bad times.

God WAS answering my prayers, but I was so caught up with anything negative, that I didn't recognize it at the time.

Codependency

During therapy I became aware that I struggled with codependency. I struggled with the need for constant reassurance for my feelings of unworthiness. I was always the one people came to when they had a problem, yet they were never around when I really needed someone. I felt empty, unfulfilled, and I lived waiting for the other shoe to drop. I yearned for a safe place to fall.

My whole life I was always over protective of my sister Tracy. I often put myself physically in front of her to protect her from my parents or anyone else who tried to mess with her. When she got older and had some struggles I did what I could to help her. Sending money or paying her rent. I allowed her to live with us while she tried to turn her life around. I learned the hard way that no matter how much you love someone you can't make them change until they are ready. Unfortunately some are never able to change and they pay the ultimate price with their lives.

I had zero tolerance for bullies in school. Often speaking up for anyone who was being victimized. I now understand that it was easier to speak up for others than it was to speak up for myself. No one ever listened when I cried for attention or needed help. I had resigned myself to believing I was unlovable. I let people treat me poorly as a result. I tolerated behaviors that left me empty and confused. How could someone who claimed to love me treat me this way? The pattern repeated throughout my lifetime. I came to expect to be treated like crap and when it didn't happen I would grow suspicious of their motives.

After Bryon and I first met I found myself trying to get him to fight with me in some attempt to prove his love for me. I needed proof. I needed him to engage with me. To fight for our love. Early in our relationship I became antagonistic in an attempt to strike first. I would get crazy when things were going well for me. I was always waiting for the other shoe to drop. When it didn't I would become fearful, and something in me would start an argument. Crazy, but that's how it was for me and unfortunately Bryon paid the price. I figured he would grow tired of me as the other men had in my life. It was not rational. It was how I'd been programmed. It was codependency. I needed him to need me as much as I needed him.

When I looked back through my life I noticed that pattern of fighting, then making up until the next time. The craziness of the instability and constant readiness to flee. Chaos... constantly. Life was exhausting. The need to please others caused me to lose sight of myself. I wanted to be indispensable. I wanted to fix things for everyone because that kept me from focusing on me. I could see everyone else's faults and felt that I knew how to fix things, yet I didn't have a clue of how to fix myself.

For years I took care of my grandma, sister, friends, father-in-law, etc., leaving no time to address myself. When my health took a hit after the cardiac arrest, I became reliant on Bryon for everything. Physically ill, mentally destroyed, and confused by the fact that I had no memory made me dependent on Bryon and anger set in. I became a victim of an unhealthy body, mind, and spirit. Anger for my circumstance kept me stuck. I was a victim of poor health. A victim of life. Dependence on alcohol no longer filled the void. I eliminated my crutches of alcohol and cigarettes. Boundaries were established and my behaviors and beliefs were challenged.

Once I understood codependency I could take steps to become more independent and I did just that. I addressed my health issues one by one. Quit drinking and smoking cigarettes. One less thing I needed Bryon to provide for me. I started to exercise to lose weight and feel better about myself. I gained energy and stamina. Clothes fit better and started to have more self confidence. I took a part time job and enjoyed having my own money again. I started setting goals and achieving them. I grew more confident in myself and my capabilities. I let go of the need to control things and I allowed myself to take risks. I surrendered my life to God and asked for guidance. I took my codependency issues back and surrendered them to God. I used to fear being alone. I now understand that I am never alone because God has been with me throughout my journey. Being codependent meant living with constant fear. I felt as if

I needed someone to always take care of me. It was a horrible way to live. Today I believe in myself. I am a divine child of God. I am on a mission to testify about what God has done for me. I have a purpose. I know that I am a strong and empathetic woman. I don't fear judgment. I live enthusiastically with eager anticipation of what will come next. Whatever it is, I know it will be great! Either a great story or a great lesson, I am up for either!

Codependency meant relying on someone other than myself for love. The solution for codependency was loving myself. Taking ownership of my life and living it as God would want me to. Being of service to others is the answer. Today I love my life. I give all the glory to God. I have gone from someone who didn't believe in myself to someone who is achieving her dreams. I am codependent no more and fully empowered with faith for the future.

Codependency meant relying on someone other than myself for love. The solution for codependency was loving myself.

How do you make healthy relationships?

When I surrendered myself to God I agreed to follow His lead. I do that by believing and following the thoughts that are my intuition. I grew up hearing it called women's intuition. It truly is a gift of guidance. It rarely leads me astray. The one time I ignored the guidance was when I met Charles. Something inside me tried to warn me, but I refused to heed the warning. I ended up paying dearly for it. These days I listen to my gut. If I meet someone and my radar alerts me to beware, I listen. My intuition is pretty spot on these days. Sobriety makes it easy to get a read on people. It has kept me safe so far. I trust God and His plan for me.

The most unexpected gift from the universe has been my new friends. The loneliness that overtook my world during recovery has been lifted. It has been replaced with meaningful relationships with people who share similar beliefs with me. Emptiness has been replaced with people who empower and believe in me and my dreams. The naysayers and phony friends have fallen by the wayside. I have a tribe of women now who I adore. Each of them is strong and courageous in their own way. I appreciate all that they bring into my life. It feels amazing to be able to share ideas about ways to help our world become a better, more compassionate place. We support each other in achieving our dreams. There is no backstabbing or gossip, just love and empathy for each other. We are all learning from one another. Sisters united to help encourage one another during difficult times in our lives. Whether it's new moms looking for advice about their children or women starting up new business endeavors, we support each other by sharing our stories and support.

I love the relationships that I have with people today. That is in large part due to the fact that I am now able to be authentically me. I live with integrity every day. I realized that by being everything to everybody, I was never actually able to be myself. I used to be worried that if I was myself people wouldn't love me. My fear of rejection kept me paralyzed for years. Now because of my relationship with God, I know that I am enough as I am. By loving myself, I am able to give love and acceptance to others. The friendships I am forming today are built on authenticity. I no longer feel like I have to prove anything to anyone anymore. I understand that we are all one energy. We are literally the vibration of energy. As humans we were designed by our creator to be a part of a larger community. We are not meant to be alone. Together we create the whole. We each have a specific way of contributing to our communities. We must understand that each of us has a unique story that makes us who we are.

God gave each of us free will and the ability to change our lives. Taking ownership of my faults and making little changes to improve my life has been very fulfilling. I am now able to help others to do the same. I am not perfect, but I have a willing heart and that is good enough for me these days. I love helping others. My job as a caregiver is also very rewarding. I wake each day with gratitude for God healing me so I can be of service to others.

I treat my clients as if they were my family members. I extend grace and compassion to them. I realize that each of us has a story. People are dealing with their own journeys so I remind myself to be kind. If I have nothing nice to say I say nothing. I am working on becoming a better listener. I acknowledge that I am a work in progress. I identify as a beautiful disaster. I am proud of everything I have been through. It's made me who I am today.

I encourage people to look inward and discover who they really are. To heal their baggage to become the best version of themselves. I surround myself with like minded people. People who care about others. People who have the courage to do the work and heal from their own BS.

While not fun to go through, the other side is so fulfilling. I admire those who are sharing their stories to give others hope.

I appreciate the little things these days. I relish having a cup of coffee with friends to catch up or a call to share exciting news. I am there for my friends through the good and bad. Always available to lend an ear to a friend who is struggling. I am grateful for my new friendships. I give God the glory because I understand all of this was by His design. He opened my eyes that my beliefs needed to be reevaluated. Now I clearly see His love for us. I live my life wanting to please Him by being a friend to others. He has given me discernment for when I meet new people so I no longer worry about getting hurt again. I do not live in fear any longer for He has blessed me with brothers/sisters in Christ. My heart is overflowing these days. I am thankful and grateful to God every morning I open my eyes.

I accept imperfection, everyone has their own story – don't get hung up on small details. I also follow my gut. I'm more in tune, more mindful of my intuition. If I feel something is off, I look into it more before judging. People can't lie to me because I can detect if they are not telling the truth. I'm more apt to look "inward" – for both me *and* them. This makes me a lot more understanding and empathetic. Though I'm still guarded with new relationships. In the end I usually find that my gut was right all along. More compassion for people. More mindfulness.

Be Kind

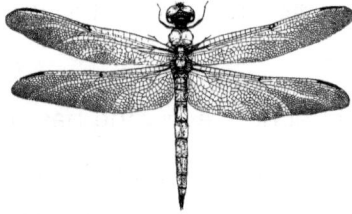

I've learned a lot from being kind. Everyone has a story. Everyone is dealing with things you are unaware of. All my life I have lived by the Golden Rule. My grandma was raised in a Catholic orphanage and later became a nun. She was a stable influence in my life. She would encourage me to walk around in others shoes before passing any judgment. Perhaps that is why I am so empathetic towards others today.

When I see someone who is struggling I immediately want to help if I can. I ask myself what I can do to remedy their situation. I believe it is what Jesus wants us to do. Grandma taught me to help whenever I can – both humans and animals.

As a child I was always rescuing stray animals. I have brought home so many over the years that I have lost track of exactly how many. I have taken in neonates or baby kittens and bottle reared them to ensure they would have the best shot at life. I have always had a natural understanding with animals. I feel their energy and I can usually comfort them when they are hurt or scared.

I have helped people in need by volunteering at the food pantry for years. I loved helping those who were truly in need. I witnessed others who were raised using it as a way to support their families for generations. I have learned not to judge any of them. I do not know their stories. I treat each of them as Jesus commands us to.

I have taken in people too that needed help. With Bryon, I cared for my grandma for 16 years, my father-in-law, and Bryon's best friend during his journey with lung cancer. I also allowed my sister and a family friend to live with us, too. I enjoy being a caregiver as a profession nowadays. I guess that is what God had been preparing me for throughout my life.

These days I understand that the only person fit to judge is Jesus. I am here to remind others of His Golden Rule, not to condemn anyone. It is my desire to remind people to just be kind.

When I was at my lowest and struggling just to get through my days, a phone call from a friend was all I needed to lift my spirits. A "thinking of you" card literally meant the world to me. It stopped me from contemplating ending my life that day. You never know what a little gesture might mean to someone. I am grateful to my friends for checking in on me when I was sick and depressed. Please do the same for the people you care about in your life. It really does make a big difference.

During the solitude of my recovery I kept getting a message of "good friend" in my mind. After the death of my best friend's mother, her father became ill with broken heart syndrome. Wanting to help I said, "we need to find your dad a friend to help him out." That's when the Papa app popped up on my phone asking if I wanted to make a difference in someone's life that day. I applied and was hired to become a Papa pal! I would become a "pal" to others in need of a friend.

This "good friend" message was actually my purpose in life. I have now been a professional caregiver for three years. I love my job. I do simple tasks that bring others joy. I spread kindness to those who need it desperately, our seniors. By being of service to others I stay busy and out of my head. Better yet, my clients have filled the void left by the death of my family members. My life has worked out for the best by listening to my inner voice, or guidance.

Surrendering my life to God has given me purpose through servitude. Learning what God wants from us is for us to be kind to one another. There is enough cruelty and evil around. Be different. Treat others as you want them to treat you. You will be surprised at how a smile at someone can brighten their dreary and predictable lives. A compliment to someone might be just what that person needs to get through their day. It doesn't take much effort, yet it can be so rewarding. Kindness truly is the best way to live your life.

My mother used kindness as a manipulation technique. She would be nice and generous during the times she had money and then she would use it to her advantage at a later time. I saw her do it, multiple times. Anytime she would offer to help me out in some way I would immediately grow suspicious of her true intentions. One must be aware of that possibility as well. I choose to be kind regardless. When I do something for someone there are no strings attached. I do it because God would want me to not because of what I can get out of it.

How does being empathic work?

When I was growing up I always felt different than others. I never understood why. When I was young I remember people engaging with my father. They admired his baseball career and usually wanted his autograph or to hear about his career highlights. He would talk to anyone. We were constantly moving around when he was traded to different teams. It caused us to be able to make new friends easily. We had no choice.

Making friends came naturally to me. I quickly learned who had good energy and who didn't. I understand now that I am a highly sensitive person, also known as an empath.

As a child I always tended to gravitate to the underdogs, always wanting to help others who are sad or struggling. That continued to the countless stray animals I could not turn away from to the tendency to want to rescue people. I have learned that rescuing isn't my job. I cannot fix those who are unwilling to take steps to change themselves. I could never get my parents to stop drinking or smoking cigarettes. I repeatedly tried to help my sister. She tried to get sober and start her life over. She wanted to be a good mother to her boys. I was sober at the time, so she was not allowed to drink while living with us. She was doing remarkably well. She found a job. We got her an apartment close to her job. I was elated to have my sister back. She was the sweetest person when she was sober. Unfortunately it didn't last long before she got in the bike wreck. All the work we had done for her didn't matter, it was over, she returned to Georgia and she died alone.

While I could never help my family I realized I had taken on their ancestral trauma and sadness. Their deaths also brought me great despair. Grief beyond anything I had ever imagined. I pleaded for death myself because I felt so lonely and abandoned. Because of my empathy for others I couldn't take my life, because of the mess that would befall to my children and husband. I had to end this generational trauma cycle in my family. I prayed for strength. I challenged God to end my pain. I begged him to take me home. I surrendered my will to God, challenging him to show me what to do with my life.

God revealed my purpose to me. He showed me that I was a good friend and caregiver.

What happened in my surrender blew my mind. I felt an instant sense of relief. I felt lighter, like I could breathe freely. Then I came to understand that this was what God had been waiting for. God is waiting for us to acknowledge Him. Because he gives us free will He waits for us to turn to Him.

After I surrendered myself to Him I had this "knowing/ understanding" of what to do next.

God revealed my purpose to me. He showed me that I was a good friend and caregiver. He created me to be an empath. I can feel others' energies. I now understand that I had gone through all the things I did so that I could help others through their difficulties. God wanted me to befriend those who were lonely and unable to stand up for themselves. To testify about the miracles that God has brought into my life. I would become a storyteller and motivator. I would share the things I had endured and that in turn would help encourage others to investigate their own relationship with their higher power. I would lead them to God.

I started journaling at the advice of my therapist. My life stories started to come to me in rhyme. Poems were flooding my mind. They weren't half bad either. I published a couple books of poems and started to give them to people. Some readers were so moved they reached out to me in gratitude. They shared their stories. I developed friendships to fill the void of friends I had lost over the years. God was bringing me new friends and opportunities to tell my story. I started healing. My depression was lifted. My love of God has filled my heart with joy. I am forever grateful for God's mercy and grace. I gained wisdom through the darkness and the struggles. God showed me that I was resilient and stronger than I ever knew. My prayers were answered. God is real. Love is real. God is love.

Being a caregiver for seniors and people with disabilities is the most rewarding thing I have ever done. I have seen some of the most tragic scenarios. I witness others who struggle with loneliness and despair. Today I am able to help them. Whether I'm cleaning their house or sitting playing cards with them, I am able to share my joy with them. It keeps me out of my head. On days when I am sad or melancholy I remind myself of how far I have come. I am proud that the generational curse has been broken. Grateful that God intervened repeatedly throughout my life so that I can be here today.

As an empath I have to limit my exposure to the news. The chaos and suffering of the world affects me deeply. God shows us what is going on so that we are aware of the devil's actions. If we are able to help bring about change we are asked to do so. We are not to turn a blind eye to suffering and corruption. Instead, we are asked to pray to God for his mercy and grace. Then we should release the negativity to the universe and practice gratitude. We must ask ourselves what we can do to help others. To be of service in our communities. To live an honorable life with integrity. It really is that simple. God wants us to be happy. We must be mindful of Him and grateful for what we have. When you emit gratitude, the universe will give you more to be grateful for. Yet if you constantly complain or focus on negativity the universe will respond negatively. If you want to be loved, give love. If you want friendship, be a friend. It's the crazy Law of Attraction in action. The Golden Rule brought to life. I dare you to give it a try. I was a nonbeliever once too.

Servitude

Since my surrender to Jesus, I have been living a life of servitude. I have recognized that I have the ability to bring joy to others. Every day I wake up eager to visit my clients. I know they enjoy these visits as much as I do. I enjoy talking to them about what's happening in my life. I share vegetables from my garden and talk about healthy recipes. I do housework that they can no longer do for themselves. It makes me feel loved and needed. I know it is what Jesus wants me to do. I have new friends now who have become like family to me. I do what I can to make their lives a little easier. As an empath I understand their loneliness and the loss of loved ones. We bring comfort to one another. I share my stories of depression. I relay how Jesus replaced my depression with purpose. I tell them how servitude helped to pull me out of my darkness and gave me hope. I no longer need to self medicate. I don't fear the feelings I get off of others. I ask myself if this emotion is really mine? Most of the time it's not. My empathy gives me a sort of insight into their world. It helps me to relate to what they might be dealing with. Then I can help them to handle whatever it is that they are experiencing. Often I share how I came to know Jesus and understand His love for us. I have never been happier in my life. I am grateful for the ability to relate to others. To understand what it feels like to walk in someone else's shoes. I am grateful for my relationship with Jesus. He is truly a miracle worker. He turned this sinner into someone who loves spreading His word and doing good for others. Glory to God.

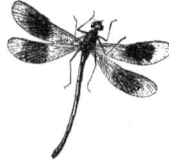

Thankful For You

We made it through another year.
Thirty two years; a reason for cheer.

I am so grateful for that fateful night.
When our eyes met; I was filled with delight.

We talked all night, until the sun rose.
We shared our stories; our tales of woe.

The connection between us was so strong.
I followed my intuition and prayed I wasn't wrong.

You were the hero I needed to heal.
My knight in shining armor; I prayed you were real.

Now it's over thirty years later and here we are.
You made my life worthwhile; glad we've made it this far!

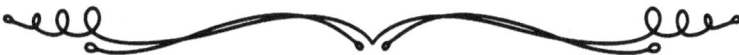

Constantly Learning

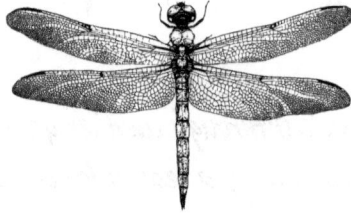

I am amazed at all that I do not know about life. Recently I was working with my clients, writing this book, and going through my day filling the hours. I could see the results of all my hard work finally starting to pay off. I am eager to be doing a storytelling presentation next month on resilience. I was speaking with the ladies involved in this presentation and learned that I was expected to speak for 30 minutes. My current story is about 10 minutes long. In my daily devotion, I relayed this worry to God. I asked him to help me to speak effectively about my resilience. I think he understood it to mean I needed another lesson in resilience. God certainly knows His stuff. He gave me one heck of a reminder of my resilience recently.

I started to feel poorly and chalked it up to overworking. My hips became stiff and uncomfortable, so I pushed harder.

Determined to do things my way. I would work as hard as I could until I couldn't. That's the kinda hard head I am. No excuses, stubbornness epitomized, I do things my way remember? So God pushed back harder. Having pushed through hip pain, now came arm, wrist, and shoulder pain and stiffness. For added measure let's throw in loss of sleep from discomfort to really get my attention. Guess who's back? Your old friend PMR. Ready to go through this again? Steroids, moonface, and massive weight gain. Remember all that you worked so hard on lately: gone. Welcome back Prednisone. Did you not understand the previous lesson? See how quickly things can change overnight? I got the message loud and clear!

I needed to be humbled. And I am thankful for the reminder. I realized I had gotten caught up in telling MY story, working on MY book, helping MY clients that I had been neglectful to God. I had made my storytelling about ME instead of God. I was proud of myself. I had become so focused on the destination that I was forgetting about enjoying the journey and being grateful for each day. I had become so distracted by his abundance in my life that I forgot to practice gratitude. I repented to Him. It wasn't just an I'm sorry Father forgive me. It was more like Please Father forgive me as the imperfect person that I am. I hear you Father and I promise to be more humble. I then asked Him to remove the symptoms of PMR from my life. I prayed that He would forgive my oversight and I promised I would be more mindful of Him. I was truly afraid I would have to take steroids and endure the nasty side effects. I worried about becoming dependent on the healthcare system again. I pleaded for His grace once more in my life. I cried myself to sleep. I awoke this morning with much less pain; this afternoon my pain has subsided completely. God answered my prayers once again. God loves each of us with our shortcomings. He is forgiveness, love, and understanding. He just wants to be acknowledged in our lives. He awaits the invitation. Be mindful that he is with us always. Lean on your faith. I encourage everyone to look inward and develop a relationship with their higher self. It might surprise even the toughest nonbeliever.

God has helped me overcome many things in my life. For instance, when I had my cardiac arrest, God gave me a second chance at life. I was blue lipped and lifeless when my husband found me. I had gone without oxygen for an unknown period of time. When I was revived by the EMTs, I was temporarily blind and had no short term memory. In the hospital I repeatedly asked my husband what time it was every minute on the minute for hours. He asked the doctor if I would ever be normal again. The prognosis was uncertain. I realize that I am blessed to be able to share my story today with others 21 years later.

God was with me through my many medical adventures. For two years before the cardiac arrest I was told that the pain I was feeling in my chest was nothing more than a panic attack.

I actually started to believe I was losing my mind. I had been prescribed antidepressants, anti-psychotics, mood stabilizers, and benzos. I had a specialist for almost every body area including heart, lungs, and liver. I epitomized illness. Fat, out of shape, addicted to meds, booze, and TV. I avoided mirrors because seeing myself literally made me sick.

I had a heart attack in my doctor's office (how perfect is that?) that resulted in two stents. Another time I developed a severe infection following a skin removal surgery four months post-op. I was very sick. I developed high fevers and my whole body was weak. They discovered two types of bacteria deep inside my upper belly just before Christmas requiring emergency surgery. God got me through it before the infection reached my bloodstream. I sustained a nasty scar which is now like a badge of honor for surviving the ordeal.

God gifted me with resilience. Each of the events in my life that caused me stress or worry was actually a lesson in the making. Resilience is a process of doing things again and again until we understand the lesson. For instance, when I was younger I kept falling for the same kinds of men. I chose older men, needing some father-type figure to take care of me. I found myself in abusive relationships time after time. I allowed them to hurt me repeatedly. Always forgiving them ,thinking there was something terribly wrong with *me*. I always felt disposable. Like something that was tossed aside when the novelty wore off.

I have learned to give myself grace. We only know what we know. We are so much more than what we are limited to in our human forms. We are energy and vibration at the very basic core of our existence. Being human is a gift. As humans we get to experience love and loss and all the emotions and feelings in between. It's an amazing journey and should be treated as such. I no longer waste my time with negativity. If I find myself going down the path of negativity I try to correct that way of thinking and look for the lessons that could be learned from the situation. When I'm feeling poorly these days I ask myself how I can remedy the situation. What can I control or do to make it better? Am I doing things to provide me with validation or am I leading them to God? God will help you too. One must surrender themselves to God. We must acknowledge that we need His guidance and Grace. Then watch what happens.

Once you acknowledge what you are, you can take steps to heal. It is OUR responsibility for self care – we must take back ownership of our own healing. Western, Eastern, whatever we need to find what is best for us.

God has brought different people into my life for me to learn from them... Sometimes I don't understand why people chose the lifestyle they do, but I am grateful that I don't need much, and realize I don't really want that "glitter."

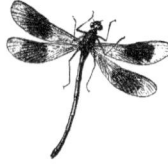

To Get Through the Day

I see you sitting over there.
I cry for you because I care.

You may be lonely, but you're not forgotten.
You must not give up even though you feel rotten.

Life changes over the years.
Our imaginations tend to amplify our fears.

People are rushing through their lives.
Sometimes it's hard just being alive.

There are some difficult lessons in life to learn.
Look to Jesus when you don't know where to turn.

He will show you the way.
Lean on Him to get through the day.

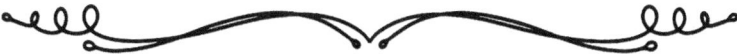

Conclusion

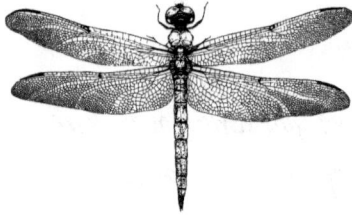

I have gone through a metamorphosis during my sobriety and spiritual awakening. Faith in something greater than myself led me to my relationship with God. Today I live in the present moment of each day. I appreciate those who have endured this process with me. Those who haven't, I wish them well too.

The changes in myself and my thought patterns are profound. I hardly remember the struggles I have endured. I choose to focus on the positives. I had to completely change my way of thinking about things. I had to question my beliefs and embrace new ideas. I had to challenge myself to learn new things. I discovered new hobbies and friends along my journey.

I had to be completely honest with myself about my role in these struggles. I had to take ownership of my shortcomings and take the steps necessary to change. I made apologies to those I had harmed. I forgave those who hurt or betrayed me. Most of all I forgave myself for not knowing better. I have learned that acknowledgment is key in taking control of my life. Once I acknowledged my faults I could take baby steps to do better. Over time I have become more patient with myself and others.

I always prayed for the life I have today. Beyond my dream of being a mom has been fulfilled, I have sons who love spending time with me. I also have a husband who adores and spoils me. I have the stability I have always needed thanks to Bryon. He is my rock. He completes me. I admit I am a handful. I had always had a reckless streak about me. The soul of a gypsy. With age I am now embracing peace instead of excitement. I no longer need to run away from myself. My soul has been restored by God's never ending love.

When I was at my lowest and bedridden with desperation and sadness it was God who saved me. When I cried out for Him to take me home He answered with I'm not finished with you. Finding my purpose was the answer. Understanding that God wants each of us to thrive and be happy. The world we are living in is filled with evil – it is Satan's world. If we turn to Jesus and repent an amazing life will unfold. It did for a sinner like me! He can help you too. Just ask Him into your heart.

My life was a complete mess for a long time. Fear of the unknown kept me paralyzed. Depression controlled my every thought and action. I now understand that depression is merely anger turned inward on oneself. My physical health was horrible. A liver mass, nodules throughout my lungs, a heart condition, or a couple of autoimmune conditions could not keep me from God's plans for me. My mental health was at its lowest after the deaths of my family members. The immense loss was unbearable for me. My immense sadness had me retreating to my cave where I literally shut down as I prayed for my end.

I was filled with rage and I wanted revenge for those who had hurt me, but God replaced rage with forgiveness and set me free. He filled my heart with love and joy. Something that I believed I was not destined to have. The gift of purpose broke the chains of depression. These days I spread love and joy to the clients I serve. My heart is full and my life is good.

I have also formed a better relationship with myself. The dialogue I have with myself is more loving and understanding as well. I have made peace with myself. Something I wish I would've done earlier. I was my own worst critic. I rode myself about everything. Believing I was fat, ugly, and worthless. My insecurities led me to self hatred and loathing. I would never have talked to anyone like I talked to myself. When I finally realized it, I took steps to make sure I never did it again. It was a slow process to love and forgive myself. No, it wasn't easy. God gave me the time I needed to figure myself out. I make the most of each day now.

In my surrender to God my life has been changed completely. I understand that we are truly living amongst evil in this world. With God in our lives we don't have to be affected by it. We can lean on God's rules and have a beautiful life despite Satan. Our faith can sustain us. Focus on the good things everyday and practice gratitude. Do unto others as you would have done to you. Be kind and helpful when you are able. It truly is that simple.

Dance of the Dragonfly is a reminder that it's up to us to take responsibility for our lives. To fix ourselves to become the best versions of ourselves and above all to keep reaching for the heavens to strengthen our relationship with God. We cannot succumb to our difficulties. It is in the darkness that we begin to grow. He wants us to lean on Him. All we need to do is to believe in ourselves. He's already given us all the tools we need in the Bible. Life is a journey of lessons. There is so much to learn. Stay curious. Look for the glimmers.

Each of us is made in God's perfect image. Everything has a reason. God thought of literally everything. I think we should all be like dragonflies. Let's take risks and step out of our comfort zones, in search of something greater in our quest for everlasting life in Heaven. We will step away from the chaos and madness in our quest for peace. We will become better versions of ourselves in the process. *Dance of the Dragonfly* is a reminder to never give up and to always believe in yourself.

About the Author

Danielle Ehlert lives in the small town of Arena, Wisconsin, with her husband Bryon and son Jake. She is also the proud mother of Brody and Bryon Jr. Danielle has called Arena home since 1993.

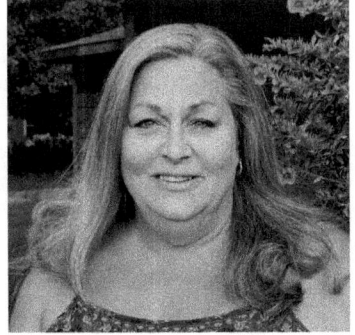

Born in 1968 during the height of her father Steve Barber's major league baseball career, Danielle was handed to her grandmother at six weeks old after her grandfather's passing. What followed was a childhood marked by abandonment, trauma, and abuse – experiences that led to lifelong emotional and physical struggles.

At 35, Danielle survived cardiac arrest. Relying on alcohol and anxiety medications to numb painful memories, she later began the hard work of healing through therapy, sobriety, and self-compassion. Battling body dysmorphia, anxiety, and grief after deep family loss, she ultimately surrendered to God – and everything changed.

Today, Danielle is a private caregiver, poet, and storyteller. Her work advocates for greater empathy and change in how society and the healthcare system treat people with mental health and addiction. Vulnerable and honest in her words, she shares her story to help others see the value in healing, and in themselves.

Visit her website: **danielleehlert.com**
to read her inspirational blog posts and check for
her lived-experience storytelling availability.

If you want to contact Dani, email her at **dani@danielleehlert.com**

www.ingramcontent.com/pod-product-compliance
Lightning Source LLC
Chambersburg PA
CBHW070108030426
42335CB00016B/2066